I0704313

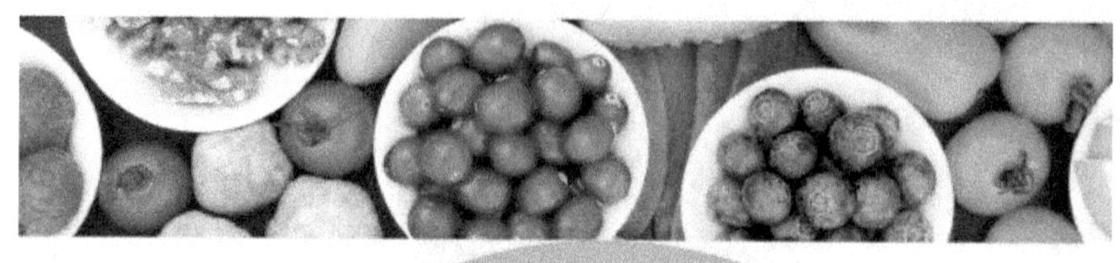

EAT TO HEAL

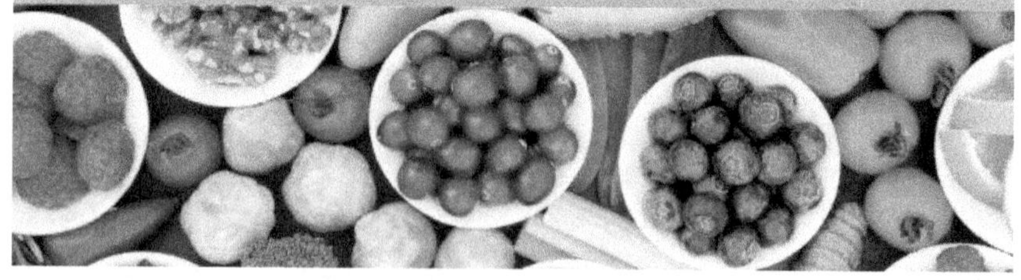

Eat to Heal: The Power of Food as Medicine for Lasting Wellness

Written by: Dr Caroline Russell

Contents

Introduction...7

  The Healing Power of Food 7

    How Food Heals...7

Part 1: The Science of Food and Healing 14

Chapter 1 15

  The Body's Natural Healing Mechanisms..15

    Understanding How Your Body Repairs and Restores Itself.............................15

  Nutrients Critical for Healing: 17

    Common Misconceptions about Food and Health..19

Chapter 2 21

  Food as Medicine: The Science Explained 21

    Nutrient-Dense Foods and Their Healing Benefits...21

  Gut Health and Its Impact on the Body 26

Chapter 3 30

  The Impact of Food on Chronic Illness...30

    How Poor Nutrition Can Lead to Disease 30

Part 2: Creating Your Healing Diet..38

Chapter 4 39

  The Healing Plate: What to Eat for Optimal Health 39

    Understanding Macronutrients: Fats, Carbs, and Proteins 39

Chapter 5 48

  Foods to Avoid: What's Harming Your Body..48

    Highly Processed Foods and the Damage They Cause 48

Chapter 6 56

  Healing Your Gut: The Key to Whole-Body Wellness...56

    Understanding the Gut Microbiome 56

    Probiotics and Prebiotics: Foods to Feed Your Gut..58

    Healing Leaky Gut Syndrome: Diet Strategies to Repair the Gut Lining 62

Chapter 7 64

  Hydration and Healing 64

    The Importance of Water for Healing and Detoxification 64

Part 3: Healing Through Different Life Stages and Conditions 71

Chapter 8 72

  Healing Foods for Common Health Issues..72

    Managing Chronic Inflammation Through Diet...72

Chapter 9 81

   Special Diets for Healing 81

      Healing with the Mediterranean Diet 81

Chapter 10 91

   Eating to Heal During Different Life Stages 91

      Nutritional Needs for Healing in Children and Adolescents 91

      Healing Foods for Women: Pregnancy, Menopause, and Beyond ... 93

Part 4: Putting Healing into Practice 99

Chapter 11 100

   Meal Planning for Healing 100

   How to Create a Healing Meal Plan: Step-by-Step Guide 100

Chapter 12 109

   Healing Recipes 109

   Breakfasts to Heal and Energize: Smoothies, Bowls, and More 109

Chapter 13 120

   Detox and Reset: The Power of Cleansing Foods 120

   Gentle Detoxification: Using Foods to Cleanse Your System 120

Chapter 14 127

   The Healing Mindset: Combining Nutrition with Lifestyle Changes 127

   The Importance of Sleep, Stress Management, and Physical Activity 127

Part 5: Sustainable Healing 134

Chapter 15 135

   Navigating the Modern Food Environment 135

   How to Choose Healing Foods at Restaurants and Social Events. 135

Chapter 16 140

   Overcoming Challenges in Your Healing Journey 140

   Dealing with Cravings and Emotional Eating 140

   The Transformative Power of Food: Recap of Key Takeaways 146

Appendices 152

   Appendix A: Comprehensive Food Lists for Healing 152

   Appendix B: Supplement Recommendations to Enhance Healing 153

   Appendix C: Glossary of Nutritional Terms and Concepts 154

References 156

Introduction

The Healing Power of Food

Food is more than just fuel for your body—it's one of the most powerful tools for healing and maintaining optimal health. Every bite you take has the potential to either contribute to your well-being or undermine it. The concept of "food as medicine" isn't new; it has roots in ancient cultures like Traditional Chinese Medicine (TCM) and Ayurveda, where diet is central to healing. Today, modern science supports this notion with extensive research on how the nutrients in our food can prevent, manage, and even reverse chronic diseases.

How Food Heals

- **Nutrient-Dense Foods:** Certain foods, like leafy greens, berries, nuts, seeds, and fatty fish, are packed with vitamins, minerals, antioxidants, and anti-inflammatory compounds. These nutrients help the body repair tissues, combat oxidative stress, and reduce inflammation.

- **Phytochemicals and Antioxidants:** These naturally occurring compounds, found in colorful fruits and vegetables, have been shown to fight cancer cells, slow the aging process, and protect the body from environmental toxins.

    - **Example:** Dark leafy greens like kale and spinach contain antioxidants such as lutein and zeaxanthin, which protect against vision-related issues like cataracts and macular degeneration.

- **Healthy Fats:** Omega-3 fatty acids, found in fish like salmon and flaxseeds, support brain health and reduce inflammation, a key driver of many chronic illnesses such as arthritis, heart disease, and diabetes.

    - **Example:** Consuming a daily portion of walnuts or flaxseeds can reduce inflammatory markers in the blood, promoting heart and brain health.

How Food Can Harm

- **Processed Foods and Inflammation:** Foods high in trans fats, refined sugars, and artificial additives can trigger chronic inflammation, which is linked to conditions like obesity, heart disease, and Alzheimer's.

    - **Example:** Regular consumption of processed foods like packaged snacks, sugary beverages, and fast food can lead to insulin resistance, promoting weight gain and increasing the risk of Type 2 diabetes.

- **Toxic Load from Pesticides and Additives:** Chemical residues on non-organic fruits and vegetables, as well as artificial sweeteners and preservatives, can disrupt the gut microbiome, weakening immunity and leading to digestive disorders.

    - **Solution:** Choose organic produce whenever possible and opt for whole, minimally processed foods to reduce your exposure to these toxins.

Why Diet Matters: A Look at Modern Health Issues

The rise of chronic diseases like obesity, diabetes, heart disease, and cancer is closely linked to poor dietary habits. Our modern food environment often promotes unhealthy choices, with ultra-processed foods, refined sugars, and unhealthy fats becoming staples in many diets. These foods not only provide little nutritional value but actively contribute to inflammation and disease.

The Global Health Crisis:

- **Obesity Epidemic:** According to the World Health Organization (WHO), global obesity rates have nearly tripled since 1975. Poor dietary choices, combined with sedentary lifestyles, are driving this epidemic.

  - **Solution:** A diet rich in whole foods, such as vegetables, fruits, lean proteins, and healthy fats, can help reverse obesity by balancing hormones, reducing inflammation, and promoting satiety.

- **Diabetes and Insulin Resistance:** Over 400 million people worldwide are affected by diabetes, largely due to the overconsumption of sugary foods and refined carbohydrates.

  - **Example:** A diet high in fiber from sources like oats, legumes, and vegetables can help stabilize blood sugar levels and reduce the risk of developing Type 2 diabetes.

The Role of Inflammation in Disease

- **Chronic Inflammation:** Inflammation is the body's natural response to injury or infection, but when it becomes chronic, it can damage healthy cells and tissues, leading to diseases like rheumatoid arthritis, cardiovascular disease, and even cancer.

    - **Example:** Chronic inflammation is often fueled by a diet high in processed meats, sugary drinks, and refined carbohydrates. However, incorporating anti-inflammatory foods like turmeric, ginger, and leafy greens can help combat this.

- **Gut Health and Disease:** The health of your gut microbiome plays a crucial role in your overall well-being. An unhealthy diet can disrupt the balance of good bacteria in the gut, leading to digestive disorders, weakened immunity, and mental health issues like anxiety and depression.

    - **Solution:** Eating a diet rich in fiber from vegetables, fruits, and whole grains, along with fermented foods like yogurt, kimchi, and sauerkraut, can support a healthy gut microbiome, boosting immunity and mood.

How This Book Will Help You Heal Naturally?

This book is designed to help you understand how the food you eat can be your most effective tool for healing. It will guide you through the science of nutrition and offer practical, actionable steps to transform your diet and improve your health. Whether you are dealing with a chronic illness or simply looking to feel better, this book provides the knowledge and resources you need to:

- **Prevent and Reverse Disease:** Learn how certain foods can reduce your risk of developing diseases like heart disease, diabetes, and cancer, and how to use food to support recovery if you're already facing health challenges.

  - **Example:** If you're dealing with high blood pressure, this book will help you understand the benefits of potassium-rich foods like bananas and spinach, which help regulate blood pressure by balancing sodium levels in your body.

- **Boost Energy and Mental Clarity:** Discover how to fuel your body with nutrient-rich foods that enhance energy levels, improve focus, and support brain health.

  - **Solution:** Adding foods rich in omega-3s, like walnuts and chia seeds, can enhance brain function, while reducing refined sugars and processed carbs can help stabilize energy levels throughout the day.

- **Enhance Digestive Health:** Get insights into foods that promote a healthy gut and improve digestion, reducing issues like bloating, constipation, and acid reflux.

  - **Solution:** Probiotic-rich foods like yogurt, kefir, and fermented vegetables can replenish the good bacteria in your gut, improving digestion and immune function.

How to Use This Guide?

A Step-by-Step Approach to Eating for Healing

This book is not just about theory—it's about practical application. Here's a step-by-step approach to using the book effectively:

1. **Start with Awareness:** Begin by understanding the importance of food in your healing journey. This includes recognizing which foods are harming your body and which can heal it.

    o **Example:** Track your current diet for a week. Note how much processed food, sugar, and artificial ingredients you're consuming. This awareness will set the foundation for making better choices.

2. **Make Gradual Changes:** You don't have to overhaul your diet overnight. Start by incorporating more healing foods into your meals, while slowly phasing out harmful options.

    o **Example:** Swap out sugary snacks for healthier alternatives like fresh fruit, nuts, or seeds. Replace processed meats with lean proteins like grilled chicken or fish.

3. **Meal Planning and Preparation:** One of the keys to a healing diet is being prepared. This book provides meal planning tips, grocery lists, and simple recipes to help you stay on track.

    o **Solution:** Use the 7-day meal plan provided in later chapters to guide your shopping and meal prep. Prepare meals in advance to make healthy eating more convenient.

4. **Stay Consistent and Listen to Your Body:** Healing with food takes time, and it's important to stay consistent. Pay attention to how your body responds as you make changes to your diet. This book will help you recognize the signs of progress and how to adjust if needed.

- o **Example:** If you notice improvements in energy levels, digestion, or mood after incorporating more whole foods, continue to build on those habits. If certain foods cause discomfort, consider removing them from your diet and consulting the elimination diet section for guidance.

By following the guidance in this book, you will learn how to take control of your health through food. You'll discover not only which foods heal but also how to make lasting dietary changes that will keep you feeling your best for years to come.

Part 1: The Science of Food and Healing

Chapter 1

The Body's Natural Healing Mechanisms

Understanding How Your Body Repairs and Restores Itself

The human body is designed to heal itself. From the moment you experience a cut or injury to more complex processes like recovering from illness, your body engages a series of automatic responses to repair damage, fight infections, and restore balance. These natural healing mechanisms are constantly at work, but they need the right environment and resources—primarily in the form of nutrients—to function optimally.

Key Healing Processes

- **Inflammation Response:**
  Inflammation is the body's first line of defense against injury or infection. When you experience a physical injury, the body sends white blood cells and immune proteins to the site of damage, causing inflammation. While short-term (acute) inflammation is beneficial, chronic inflammation is harmful, leading to long-term damage and diseases such as arthritis, cardiovascular disease, and even cancer.

  - **Example:** A cut on your skin swells and becomes red due to the inflammatory response, which helps to protect the area from infection and starts the healing process.

  - **Role of Nutrition:** Anti-inflammatory foods, such as fatty fish rich in omega-3 fatty acids (like salmon), turmeric, and leafy greens, can help regulate this process by reducing chronic inflammation.

- **Cellular Repair and Regeneration:**
  Cells in your body are constantly being damaged and replaced. Certain tissues, like skin, bone, and muscle, regenerate more quickly, while others, such as nerve cells, take longer to heal. The speed and efficiency of cellular repair depend heavily on the availability of nutrients like proteins, vitamins, and minerals.

- **Example:** The skin completely renews itself every 28-30 days, but if you're lacking essential nutrients like Vitamin A or Vitamin C, this process slows down, leaving you prone to infections or skin conditions like acne or eczema.

  - **Role of Nutrition:** Protein-rich foods (like beans, lentils, chicken), Vitamin C (found in citrus fruits), and Vitamin A (from foods like carrots and sweet potatoes) are critical for tissue repair and skin regeneration.

- **Detoxification:**

  The body is constantly detoxifying itself through organs like the liver and kidneys, which filter out harmful substances and waste products from the blood. The efficiency of this detox system can be enhanced by certain foods, while toxins from poor-quality diets (like processed foods) can burden these organs, slowing the process down.

  - **Example:** A diet rich in antioxidants, such as berries, green tea, and cruciferous vegetables (like broccoli and Brussels sprouts), supports liver function and promotes detoxification.

  - **Role of Nutrition:** Drinking plenty of water and eating fiber-rich foods (like whole grains and vegetables) helps your body flush out toxins more efficiently.

Key Takeaway:

While your body has impressive built-in mechanisms to heal, repair, and restore itself, these processes can only function optimally if you provide the right nutrients. A diet rich in vitamins, minerals, healthy fats, proteins, and antioxidants supports your body's natural ability to heal.

The Role of Nutrition in Self-Healing

Nutrition is the fuel that powers your body's healing processes. Every cell, tissue, and organ depends on the nutrients you consume to function correctly. When your diet is deficient in essential nutrients, it compromises your body's ability to repair and regenerate. Conversely, when you eat a nutrient-rich diet, you give your body the tools it needs to heal faster, fight off disease, and maintain overall health.

Nutrients Critical for Healing:

- **Proteins:**

  Proteins are the building blocks of life. They help repair damaged tissues and build new cells. Every time your body heals a wound or regenerates cells, it uses proteins derived from the food you eat.

  - **Examples of Protein Sources:** Eggs, chicken, tofu, beans, and fish.

  - **Healing Role:** If you're recovering from surgery or injury, increasing your protein intake helps speed up tissue repair.

- **Vitamins and Minerals:**

  - **Vitamin C** supports collagen production, which is essential for wound healing and skin repair.

    - **Sources:** Citrus fruits, strawberries, bell peppers.

  - **Vitamin A** plays a role in immune function and helps heal skin wounds.

    - **Sources:** Carrots, sweet potatoes, spinach.

  - **Zinc** is necessary for tissue repair, immune function, and cell division.

    - **Sources:** Pumpkin seeds, lentils, chickpeas.

  - **Magnesium** is critical for over 300 biochemical reactions in the body, including muscle recovery and relaxation.

    - **Sources:** Leafy greens, nuts, seeds, whole grains.

- **Healthy Fats:**
  Omega-3 fatty acids, found in fatty fish, flaxseeds, and walnuts, are powerful anti-inflammatory agents that reduce chronic inflammation and promote heart, brain, and joint health.

  - **Healing Role:** Omega-3s can help alleviate symptoms in conditions like arthritis by reducing inflammation and promoting joint health.

- **Antioxidants:**
  Antioxidants protect your body from oxidative stress, which occurs when free radicals (unstable molecules) damage cells. This damage plays a role in aging and the development of chronic diseases.

  - **Sources:** Blueberries, spinach, nuts, dark chocolate.

  - **Healing Role:** Antioxidants found in colorful fruits and vegetables help the body repair from oxidative damage, promoting faster recovery from illness or injury.

Real-Life Example of Healing Through Nutrition:

Imagine you've recently suffered from a cold or flu. While your body works to fight off the virus, supporting your immune system through nutrition can speed recovery. Foods rich in Vitamin C (oranges, kiwi), Zinc (nuts, seeds), and antioxidants (berries, green tea) give your immune system the boost it needs to clear the infection more quickly, reducing the length and severity of your symptoms.

Key Takeaway:

A balanced, nutrient-dense diet is essential for self-healing. Every vitamin, mineral, and macronutrient has a role to play in your body's recovery and maintenance. By incorporating these healing foods into your daily meals, you help your body perform its natural healing functions more efficiently.

Common Misconceptions about Food and Health

There is a lot of confusion surrounding the relationship between food and health, largely due to misinformation, trends, and myths perpetuated by social media, advertisements, and even some popular diets. Let's clarify some of the most common misconceptions.

1. "Calories are all that matters."

Many people believe that as long as they control their calorie intake, they can eat whatever they want and still be healthy. While maintaining a healthy weight is important, the quality of those calories is equally crucial. A diet high in processed foods, sugars, and unhealthy fats can still cause inflammation, nutrient deficiencies, and chronic diseases, even if you're not overeating.

- **Example:** 500 calories of fast food (a burger and fries) vs. 500 calories of whole foods (a salad with grilled chicken, avocado, and nuts) have drastically different effects on your health. The fast food is high in trans fats, refined carbs, and sugars that promote inflammation, while the whole foods provide vitamins, minerals, and fiber that support healing.

2. "All fats are bad."

Fat has often been demonized in mainstream diet advice, but not all fats are created equal. While trans fats and excessive saturated fats can be harmful, healthy fats like omega-3 fatty acids are essential for brain health, reducing inflammation, and supporting heart function.

- **Solution:** Instead of cutting out all fats, focus on incorporating healthy fat sources like olive oil, nuts, seeds, and fatty fish into your diet.

3. "Supplements can replace food."

While supplements can be beneficial for filling in nutrient gaps, they are not a substitute for a nutrient-dense diet. Whole foods contain a complex combination of vitamins, minerals, fiber, and other compounds that work together synergistically to support health—something that isolated supplements can't fully replicate.

- **Example:** Taking a Vitamin C supplement is not as effective as eating an orange, which also provides fiber, antioxidants, and other compounds that enhance the vitamin's absorption and impact.

4. "A 'detox' diet is necessary to cleanse your body."

Many people believe that special detox diets or juice cleanses are necessary to rid the body of toxins. In reality, your body has its own sophisticated detoxification systems (primarily through the liver, kidneys, and skin) that work continuously to eliminate waste and toxins.

- **Solution:** Rather than relying on drastic detox diets, focus on eating whole, nutrient-rich foods that support the liver and kidneys, like leafy greens, cruciferous vegetables, and plenty of water.

Key Takeaway:

While there are many myths surrounding food and health, understanding the science behind nutrition can help you make informed decisions. It's not just about calories, fats, or supplements—it's about nourishing your body with whole, nutrient-dense foods that support its natural healing processes.

The body's natural healing mechanisms are incredibly powerful, but they require the right nutrition to function effectively. By understanding how your body repairs and restores itself, and by debunking common misconceptions, you can take control of your health. Proper nutrition, rich in healing nutrients, will enhance your body's ability to fight disease, recover from injury, and maintain long-term well-being.

Chapter 2

Food as Medicine: The Science Explained

Nutrient-Dense Foods and Their Healing Benefits

Nutrient-dense foods are those that provide high levels of essential nutrients (vitamins, minerals, fiber, antioxidants) relative to their calorie content. These foods not only nourish the body but also support its ability to repair, regenerate, and fight disease. By consuming nutrient-dense foods, you enhance your body's natural healing mechanisms and prevent the onset of chronic diseases.

Top Nutrient-Dense Foods and Their Benefits

1. **Leafy Greens (e.g., spinach, kale, arugula):**

   o **Healing Benefits:** Rich in vitamins A, C, K, and folate, leafy greens are powerful antioxidants that protect the body from oxidative stress, promote healthy blood clotting, and support immune function.

   o **Example:** Spinach is particularly high in magnesium, which is essential for muscle relaxation and nervous system health.

2. **Berries (e.g., blueberries, strawberries, raspberries):**

   o **Healing Benefits:** Berries are rich in fiber, vitamins (particularly vitamin C), and antioxidants like anthocyanins, which reduce inflammation and combat cellular damage.

   o **Example:** Blueberries are known for improving brain function and protecting against age-related memory decline due to their high levels of flavonoids.

3. **Fatty Fish (e.g., salmon, mackerel, sardines):**

   o **Healing Benefits:** Fatty fish are excellent sources of omega-3 fatty acids, which reduce inflammation, support brain health, and promote heart health.

- o **Example:** Consuming omega-3-rich fish can lower the risk of heart disease by reducing triglyceride levels and improving artery function.

4. **Nuts and Seeds (e.g., almonds, flaxseeds, chia seeds):**

    - o **Healing Benefits:** These are packed with healthy fats, fiber, protein, vitamins (like vitamin E), and minerals. They reduce inflammation, improve heart health, and support cognitive function.

    - o **Example:** Almonds are a great source of vitamin E, which helps protect cells from oxidative damage and promotes skin health.

5. **Whole Grains (e.g., quinoa, oats, brown rice):**

    - o **Healing Benefits:** Whole grains are rich in fiber, which supports gut health and stabilizes blood sugar levels. They are also packed with vitamins like B-complex and essential minerals like magnesium.

    - o **Example:** Oats contain beta-glucan, a type of soluble fiber that helps reduce cholesterol levels and promote heart health.

Key Takeaway:

Focusing on nutrient-dense foods provides your body with the essential components needed for healing, cellular repair, and overall vitality. These foods help prevent and manage chronic conditions while boosting your energy, mood, and resilience to illness.

Anti-inflammatory Foods vs. Inflammatory Foods

Inflammation is a natural bodily response to injury or infection, but chronic inflammation can lead to diseases like heart disease, diabetes, and cancer. Your diet plays a significant role in either exacerbating or reducing inflammation in the body. Anti-inflammatory foods help to reduce inflammation, while inflammatory foods can fuel it.

Anti-inflammatory Foods:

1. **Turmeric:**

   - **Healing Benefits:** Curcumin, the active compound in turmeric, has powerful anti-inflammatory and antioxidant properties. It helps reduce inflammation in joints and tissues, particularly in conditions like arthritis.

   - **Example:** Consuming turmeric in combination with black pepper (which enhances curcumin absorption) can significantly reduce joint pain and swelling in people with rheumatoid arthritis.

2. **Ginger:**

   - **Healing Benefits:** Ginger contains bioactive compounds like gingerol, which reduce inflammation, particularly in the digestive system. It can help alleviate symptoms of nausea, arthritis, and digestive discomfort.

   - **Example:** Ginger tea is a natural remedy for soothing stomach aches and improving digestion after meals.

3. **Fatty Fish (Omega-3s):**

   - **Healing Benefits:** Omega-3 fatty acids found in fish like salmon and sardines reduce chronic inflammation by lowering inflammatory markers in the blood, such as C-reactive protein (CRP).

   - **Example:** Regular consumption of fatty fish has been shown to reduce the risk of chronic diseases like heart disease and rheumatoid arthritis.

4. **Berries (High in Antioxidants):**

    o   **Healing Benefits:** Rich in antioxidants, berries help neutralize free radicals, which can trigger inflammation. They also contain compounds that boost immune function and improve circulation.

    o   **Example:** Eating a daily serving of strawberries can reduce the inflammatory response in people with metabolic syndrome.

5. **Olive Oil:**

    o   **Healing Benefits:** Extra virgin olive oil contains oleocanthal, a compound with anti-inflammatory effects similar to ibuprofen. It reduces the risk of heart disease by lowering inflammatory markers.

    o   **Example:** Incorporating olive oil into your diet can reduce inflammation and improve cholesterol levels, lowering the risk of heart disease.

Inflammatory Foods:

1. **Processed and Refined Sugars:**

    o   **Impact:** Consuming high amounts of sugar spikes blood glucose levels, leading to insulin resistance and promoting inflammation. Sugary foods and beverages contribute to obesity, diabetes, and heart disease.

    o   **Example:** Soft drinks, candy, and pastries are high in sugar and can exacerbate inflammation in the body, leading to joint pain and increased risk of chronic diseases.

2. **Trans Fats (Found in Processed and Fried Foods):**

    o   **Impact:** Trans fats, found in many processed foods, increase inflammation by raising levels of LDL (bad cholesterol) and lowering HDL (good cholesterol).

    o   **Example:** Regular consumption of trans fats from foods like margarine, packaged snacks, and fried foods is linked to an increased risk of heart disease and inflammation-related disorders.

3. **Refined Carbohydrates (e.g., White Bread, Pasta, Pastries):**

   o **Impact:** Refined carbohydrates cause rapid spikes in blood sugar, leading to insulin resistance and inflammation. They lack fiber and essential nutrients, making them harmful to long-term health.

   o **Example:** White bread and pasta, when consumed in large amounts, can lead to chronic inflammation and increased risk of diabetes.

4. **Processed Meats (e.g., Bacon, Sausage, Hot Dogs):**

   o **Impact:** These meats are high in saturated fats, preservatives, and other harmful compounds like nitrates, which increase inflammation and raise the risk of heart disease and colon cancer.

   o **Example:** Frequent consumption of processed meats has been linked to higher levels of inflammatory markers, contributing to cardiovascular disease.

Key Takeaway:

Choosing anti-inflammatory foods and avoiding inflammatory ones can significantly reduce your risk of chronic diseases and improve overall health. A diet rich in whole, unprocessed foods promotes a balanced inflammatory response in the body, keeping you healthier for longer.

The Gut-Health Connection: Why Your Digestive System is Key to Healing

Your gut is more than just a system for digesting food—it is central to your overall health. A healthy gut, populated by diverse and beneficial bacteria, supports digestion, boosts immunity, regulates mood, and even influences inflammation levels throughout the body. When the gut is compromised, it can lead to issues like leaky gut, which has been linked to chronic illnesses, autoimmune diseases, and even mental health problems.

Gut Health and Its Impact on the Body

1. **Digestive Health:**

   A healthy gut ensures proper digestion and nutrient absorption. When gut health is compromised, symptoms like bloating, constipation, diarrhea, and nutrient deficiencies can occur.

   - **Example:** Fiber-rich foods like beans, lentils, and whole grains promote healthy digestion and prevent constipation.

2. **Immunity:**

   Around 70% of your immune system resides in the gut. A healthy gut microbiome can enhance immune responses, protecting the body from infections and inflammation.

   - **Example:** Fermented foods like yogurt, kefir, and sauerkraut introduce beneficial probiotics, which support immune function and reduce the risk of infections.

3. **Inflammation Regulation:**

   An imbalanced gut can trigger chronic inflammation in the body. Gut dysbiosis, where harmful bacteria outnumber beneficial ones, can contribute to diseases like irritable bowel syndrome (IBS), rheumatoid arthritis, and even depression.

o   **Example:** Consuming prebiotic foods like onions, garlic, and asparagus feeds the beneficial bacteria in the gut, promoting a healthy balance and reducing inflammation.

How to Support Gut Health?

- **Probiotic-Rich Foods:** Fermented foods such as yogurt, kimchi, kombucha, and pickles introduce beneficial bacteria that improve gut health.

- **Prebiotic Foods:** Foods high in fiber, such as garlic, onions, and bananas, act as food for the healthy bacteria in your gut, ensuring they thrive.

- **Avoid Overuse of Antibiotics:** Antibiotics can kill off beneficial bacteria along with harmful ones, leading to gut imbalances. If antibiotics are necessary, consider taking a probiotic supplement to restore healthy bacteria.

- **Limit Processed Foods and Sugar:** Processed foods and sugars promote the growth of harmful bacteria and yeast, leading to imbalances that negatively affect gut health.

Key Takeaway:

Maintaining a healthy gut is essential for overall health and healing. By incorporating gut-friendly foods, you can support digestion, strengthen immunity, and reduce inflammation, leading to better long-term health outcomes.

Phytochemicals and Antioxidants: Nature's Own Healers

Phytochemicals are naturally occurring compounds found in plants that have powerful health benefits. These compounds, along with antioxidants, protect cells from damage, fight inflammation, and help prevent chronic diseases. They work by neutralizing free radicals—unstable molecules that can cause cellular damage and contribute to diseases like cancer and heart disease.

Powerful Phytochemicals and Their Sources:

1. **Flavonoids (Found in Berries, Apples, and Citrus Fruits):**

   - **Healing Benefits:** Flavonoids have strong anti-inflammatory and antioxidant properties. They help protect the heart, reduce the risk of stroke, and support brain health.

   - **Example:** Regular consumption of flavonoid-rich foods like blueberries can improve memory and cognitive function, particularly in aging individuals.

2. **Carotenoids (Found in Carrots, Sweet Potatoes, and Tomatoes):**

   - **Healing Benefits:** Carotenoids are converted to vitamin A in the body, which supports eye health, boosts immunity, and promotes skin health.

   - **Example:** Beta-carotene, the carotenoid responsible for the orange color in carrots, is critical for maintaining healthy vision.

3. **Polyphenols (Found in Green Tea, Dark Chocolate, and Red Wine):**

   - **Healing Benefits:** Polyphenols improve circulation, reduce inflammation, and support brain health. They also help lower the risk of cardiovascular diseases.

   - **Example:** The polyphenols in green tea (such as catechins) have been shown to boost metabolism and improve heart health.

4. **Sulforaphane (Found in Cruciferous Vegetables like Broccoli, Kale, and Brussels Sprouts):**

   o **Healing Benefits:** Sulforaphane has potent anti-cancer properties and supports detoxification by enhancing the body's ability to eliminate toxins.

   o **Example:** Regular consumption of broccoli can reduce the risk of cancer and support liver function due to its high sulforaphane content.

Key Takeaway:

Phytochemicals and antioxidants are nature's own defense system, offering protection against cellular damage, inflammation, and disease. Including a variety of colorful fruits, vegetables, and plant-based foods in your diet ensures that your body receives the healing benefits of these powerful compounds.

Food is more than just fuel—it is medicine. By understanding the healing power of nutrient-dense foods, the impact of inflammation, the crucial role of gut health, and the protective properties of phytochemicals and antioxidants, you can harness the full potential of food to promote healing and prevent disease. Through mindful choices, you can nourish your body, reduce inflammation, and support long-term health.

Chapter 3
The Impact of Food on Chronic Illness

How Poor Nutrition Can Lead to Disease

Poor nutrition is a leading cause of many chronic illnesses, including heart disease, diabetes, obesity, and even some cancers. The modern diet, which is often high in processed foods, refined sugars, unhealthy fats, and low in essential nutrients, creates the perfect environment for disease to thrive. Over time, the cumulative effects of a poor diet can lead to systemic inflammation, insulin resistance, obesity, and other metabolic disorders, weakening the body's natural defense mechanisms and increasing susceptibility to illness.

Key Ways Poor Nutrition Contributes to Chronic Disease:

1. **Chronic Inflammation:**
   A diet high in processed and sugary foods promotes chronic inflammation, which is linked to various diseases like arthritis, heart disease, and cancer. Inflammatory foods, such as trans fats, refined carbohydrates, and sugary beverages, increase the production of inflammatory molecules in the body.

   o **Example:** Regularly consuming fast food meals, which are high in trans fats, can lead to persistent inflammation that damages arteries and increases the risk of heart attacks.

2. **Insulin Resistance and Type 2 Diabetes:**
   Excessive consumption of refined sugars and simple carbohydrates can cause blood sugar levels to spike frequently. Over time, this leads to insulin resistance, where the body's cells stop responding to insulin effectively. This resistance can eventually lead to type 2 diabetes.

   o **Example:** A diet rich in sugary drinks, white bread, and pastries leads to constant blood sugar spikes, forcing the pancreas to produce more insulin.

Over time, the body becomes less sensitive to insulin, leading to type 2 diabetes.

3. **Obesity and Metabolic Syndrome:**

High-calorie, nutrient-poor foods contribute to weight gain and obesity, which increases the risk of metabolic syndrome—a cluster of conditions including high blood pressure, high cholesterol, and high blood sugar that heightens the risk of heart disease, stroke, and diabetes.

- o **Example:** A daily intake of sugary sodas, fast food, and snacks like chips can contribute to weight gain, which increases the risk of developing metabolic syndrome.

4. **Heart Disease:**

Diets high in saturated fats, trans fats, and cholesterol contribute to the buildup of plaque in the arteries (atherosclerosis), which is a leading cause of heart disease. Elevated cholesterol levels, especially LDL (bad cholesterol), increase the risk of heart attacks and strokes.

- o **Example:** Regular consumption of processed meats, fried foods, and margarine leads to higher LDL cholesterol, which can clog arteries and increase the risk of cardiovascular disease.

5. **Nutrient Deficiencies:**

Poor diets often lack essential vitamins, minerals, and antioxidants that the body needs for optimal functioning. Deficiencies in key nutrients like magnesium, vitamin D, and omega-3 fatty acids can exacerbate health problems like depression, poor bone health, and cognitive decline.

- o **Example:** A diet low in leafy greens, nuts, and seeds can lead to magnesium deficiency, which is linked to muscle cramps, fatigue, and increased risk of heart disease.

Key Takeaway:

Poor nutrition doesn't just affect how you feel in the short term—it has long-lasting impacts on your body. A diet lacking in essential nutrients and full of inflammatory, processed foods paves the way for chronic illnesses to develop. By understanding how poor nutrition contributes to disease, you can begin to make informed choices that prioritize your long-term health.

Reversing the Damage: How Diet Can Improve Conditions Like Diabetes, Heart Disease, and More

The body has an incredible capacity to heal itself, even after years of poor nutrition. By making targeted dietary changes, many chronic conditions can be managed or even reversed. A whole-food, nutrient-rich diet, combined with lifestyle changes like regular physical activity and stress management, can halt the progression of many diseases and in some cases, lead to significant improvements or remission.

Conditions that Can Be Improved or Reversed Through Diet:

1. **Type 2 Diabetes:**

   - **How Diet Helps:** A diet low in refined sugars and carbohydrates, paired with an emphasis on whole foods like vegetables, lean proteins, and healthy fats, can stabilize blood sugar levels and increase insulin sensitivity. Whole foods are digested more slowly, leading to gradual blood sugar increases instead of spikes.

   - **Example:** Studies have shown that a low-carbohydrate, high-fiber diet can reduce HbA1c levels (a measure of long-term blood glucose levels) in people with type 2 diabetes, sometimes eliminating the need for medication.

   - **Solution:** Replace refined grains with whole grains, and sugary snacks with fruits, nuts, and seeds. For example, instead of a sugary cereal, choose a bowl of oats topped with chia seeds, berries, and almond butter.

2. **Heart Disease:**

   - **How Diet Helps:** A heart-healthy diet rich in omega-3 fatty acids, fiber, and antioxidants can reduce cholesterol levels, lower blood pressure, and improve overall cardiovascular health. Reducing intake of trans fats and saturated fats can help unclog arteries and reduce inflammation.

   - **Example:** The Mediterranean diet, which emphasizes olive oil, fatty fish, whole grains, and plenty of fruits and vegetables, has been shown to reduce the risk of heart disease by improving cholesterol profiles and reducing inflammation.

- o **Solution:** Incorporate more heart-healthy fats like those found in avocados, nuts, and olive oil. Replace red meats with fish like salmon or mackerel, and eat plenty of leafy greens and cruciferous vegetables like broccoli.

3. **Hypertension (High Blood Pressure):**

- o **How Diet Helps:** A diet low in sodium and rich in potassium, magnesium, and calcium can help regulate blood pressure levels. Foods like leafy greens, bananas, sweet potatoes, and legumes can naturally lower blood pressure.

- o **Example:** The DASH (Dietary Approaches to Stop Hypertension) diet has been proven to lower blood pressure by emphasizing fruits, vegetables, whole grains, lean proteins, and limiting sodium.

- o **Solution:** Reduce your intake of processed and salty foods, and increase your consumption of potassium-rich foods like bananas, oranges, and spinach.

4. **Obesity and Metabolic Syndrome:**

- o **How Diet Helps:** A balanced diet that emphasizes whole, unprocessed foods and is high in fiber, protein, and healthy fats helps regulate appetite, improve metabolism, and support healthy weight loss. Reducing refined sugars and processed carbohydrates is key to preventing blood sugar spikes that lead to fat storage.

- o **Example:** Many people find success by adopting a plant-based or low-carb diet, which helps with weight loss and reduces the risk of metabolic syndrome.

- o **Solution:** Replace high-calorie processed snacks with nutrient-dense options like nuts, seeds, and fresh vegetables. A typical high-fiber, low-sugar meal could include grilled salmon with quinoa and steamed broccoli.

5. **Autoimmune Disorders (e.g., Rheumatoid Arthritis, Lupus):**

   - **How Diet Helps:** Inflammatory autoimmune conditions can often be managed with an anti-inflammatory diet that removes common triggers like processed foods, sugars, and unhealthy fats, while including foods that reduce inflammation (such as fatty fish, nuts, seeds, and leafy greens).

   - **Example:** Studies have shown that a diet rich in omega-3s, such as from fish and flaxseeds, can reduce joint pain and stiffness in patients with rheumatoid arthritis.

   - **Solution:** Focus on eating anti-inflammatory foods such as berries, fatty fish, and turmeric, while avoiding inflammatory triggers like refined sugar and trans fats.

Real-Life Success Stories:

Many people have successfully reversed or improved their chronic conditions through diet. For example, individuals with type 2 diabetes who adopted a low-carb, high-fiber diet have reported reduced dependence on insulin and other medications, while those with heart disease have seen improvements in cholesterol and blood pressure through plant-based diets.

Key Takeaway:

The right dietary changes can make a profound difference in managing or even reversing chronic conditions. By focusing on whole foods, minimizing processed foods, and targeting specific nutrients, you can take significant steps toward healing and reducing your reliance on medications.

The Power of Prevention: Eating to Stay Healthy

While it is possible to reverse some damage caused by poor nutrition, prevention is always the best approach. By adopting a nutrient-rich, balanced diet early on, you can significantly reduce your risk of developing chronic diseases and enjoy a higher quality of life as you age. Preventative nutrition focuses on maintaining a healthy body and immune system, preventing the onset of illness, and promoting longevity.

Key Principles of a Preventative Diet

1. **Balanced Macronutrients:**

   - Eating a balanced diet that includes the right proportions of carbohydrates, proteins, and fats is essential for maintaining a healthy metabolism and preventing nutrient deficiencies. Opt for complex carbohydrates (like whole grains), lean proteins (like fish, beans, and legumes), and healthy fats (like avocado and olive oil).

   - **Example:** Instead of a refined carb-heavy meal like pasta with a cream sauce, opt for whole-grain pasta with grilled chicken and sautéed vegetables.

2. **High Fiber Intake:**

   - Fiber is critical for digestive health and helps regulate blood sugar levels, maintain a healthy weight, and lower cholesterol. Aim to get at least 25-30 grams of fiber per day from fruits, vegetables, whole grains, and legumes.

   - **Example:** Start your day with a fiber-rich breakfast like oatmeal with flaxseeds, berries, and a handful of almonds.

3. **Antioxidant-Rich Foods:**

   - Antioxidants protect your cells from damage caused by oxidative stress, which contributes to aging and chronic diseases. Eating a variety of colorful fruits and vegetables ensures that you get a wide range of antioxidants.

- o **Example:** Include a rainbow of vegetables in your meals, such as spinach, bell peppers, carrots, and beets, to maximize antioxidant intake.

4. **Hydration:**

   - o Staying hydrated is essential for every bodily function, from digestion to circulation to temperature regulation. Drinking plenty of water helps flush toxins from your body and keeps your metabolism functioning optimally.

   - o **Example:** Replace sugary drinks with water, herbal teas, or sparkling water flavored with lemon or cucumber.

5. **Minimizing Processed Foods and Sugars:**

   - o Processed foods often contain unhealthy additives like trans fats, excessive sodium, and added sugars that contribute to inflammation and chronic disease. Limiting these foods is key to maintaining long-term health.

   - o **Example:** Instead of processed snacks like chips or candy, choose whole foods like nuts, fruits, and veggies.

Key Takeaway:

Prevention is more effective than cure. By consistently making healthy food choices, you can reduce your risk of chronic illnesses and maintain good health as you age. A well-balanced, nutrient-rich diet not only prevents disease but also promotes vitality and longevity.

The foods we eat have a profound impact on our health. Poor nutrition is a major contributor to chronic diseases like diabetes, heart disease, and obesity, but the good news is that the damage can often be reversed or prevented with the right dietary changes. By understanding how nutrition affects chronic illness, making informed food choices, and prioritizing prevention, you can take control of your health and live a longer, healthier life.

Part 2: Creating Your Healing Diet

Chapter 4

The Healing Plate: What to Eat for Optimal Health

Understanding Macronutrients: Fats, Carbs, and Proteins

Macronutrients—fats, carbohydrates, and proteins—are the foundation of any diet. Each macronutrient plays a critical role in supporting your body's functions, from energy production to tissue repair. Understanding how to balance these macronutrients is key to creating a healing diet that promotes optimal health.

1. Fats: The Good, the Bad, and the Essential

Fats are essential for brain function, hormone production, and the absorption of fat-soluble vitamins (A, D, E, and K). However, not all fats are created equal. It's important to distinguish between healthy fats that promote healing and unhealthy fats that contribute to inflammation and chronic disease.

- **Healthy Fats (Monounsaturated and Polyunsaturated Fats):** These fats reduce inflammation, improve heart health, and support brain function.

    - **Sources:** Avocados, olive oil, nuts, seeds, and fatty fish like salmon.

    - **Example:** A Mediterranean-style diet rich in olive oil and nuts has been shown to reduce the risk of heart disease and stroke.

- **Unhealthy Fats (Trans Fats and Excess Saturated Fats):** These fats contribute to inflammation, raise bad cholesterol (LDL), and increase the risk of heart disease.

    - **Sources:** Processed snacks, margarine, fried foods, and high-fat meats.

    - **Example:** Studies link the consumption of trans fats, found in many baked goods and fast foods, to an increased risk of cardiovascular disease.

2. Carbohydrates: Fuel for the Body

Carbohydrates are the body's main source of energy. However, the type of carbohydrates you consume matters greatly. Simple carbohydrates (like refined sugars and white flour) cause blood sugar spikes and crashes, while complex carbohydrates provide sustained energy and essential fiber.

- **Complex Carbohydrates:** These carbs are packed with fiber, which helps stabilize blood sugar, support gut health, and reduce the risk of chronic diseases.

  - **Sources:** Whole grains (brown rice, quinoa, oats), legumes (beans, lentils), vegetables, and fruits.

  - **Example:** A fiber-rich breakfast of oatmeal with berries provides sustained energy and helps regulate blood sugar throughout the morning.

- **Simple Carbohydrates:** These are quickly digested, leading to rapid spikes in blood sugar and insulin levels, which can contribute to weight gain and insulin resistance.

  - **Sources:** Sugary snacks, white bread, pastries, and sodas.

  - **Example:** Replacing a sugary snack with a piece of fruit provides natural sugars along with fiber, vitamins, and antioxidants.

3. Proteins: The Building Blocks of Healing

Proteins are crucial for repairing tissues, building muscles, and supporting immune function. A balanced intake of protein helps maintain muscle mass, promotes healing, and supports metabolic function.

- **Complete Proteins (Containing All Essential Amino Acids):** These proteins are found in animal products and some plant-based sources.

  - **Sources:** Chicken, fish, eggs, dairy, and plant-based options like quinoa and soy products.

  - **Example:** Grilled salmon paired with quinoa provides a complete protein meal that supports muscle repair and offers heart-healthy omega-3 fatty acids.

- **Incomplete Proteins (Missing Some Essential Amino Acids):** Many plant-based proteins are incomplete but can be combined to form complete proteins.

  - **Sources:** Beans, lentils, nuts, seeds, and whole grains.

o   **Example:** A combination of rice and beans creates a complete protein, providing all essential amino acids needed for tissue repair and growth.

Key Takeaway:

Balancing fats, carbs, and proteins is essential for creating a diet that promotes healing and optimal health. By focusing on healthy fats, complex carbs, and quality proteins, you can provide your body with the fuel it needs to repair, grow, and thrive.

The Role of Micronutrients: Vitamins and Minerals for Healing

While macronutrients provide energy, micronutrients—vitamins and minerals—are essential for supporting the body's biochemical processes. Deficiencies in key micronutrients can impair healing, weaken the immune system, and lead to chronic health issues.

Key Micronutrients for Healing:

1. **Vitamin C (Ascorbic Acid):**

   o **Role:** Supports immune function, promotes collagen production (important for skin, bones, and connective tissue), and acts as a powerful antioxidant.

   o **Sources:** Citrus fruits (oranges, lemons), bell peppers, strawberries, and broccoli.

   o **Example:** Regular consumption of vitamin C-rich foods can help speed up wound healing and protect against infections.

2. **Vitamin D:**

   o **Role:** Supports bone health by regulating calcium absorption, boosts immune function, and plays a role in reducing inflammation.

   o **Sources:** Sunlight exposure, fortified foods (like milk and orange juice), fatty fish (like salmon), and egg yolks.

   o **Example:** Individuals with vitamin D deficiency are at higher risk for bone fractures and autoimmune diseases. Ensuring adequate intake supports both bone health and immune resilience.

3. **Magnesium:**

   o **Role:** Supports over 300 biochemical reactions in the body, including muscle and nerve function, blood sugar control, and energy production.

   o **Sources:** Leafy green vegetables, nuts, seeds, whole grains, and legumes.

   o **Example:** Magnesium-rich foods like spinach and almonds can help reduce muscle cramps and improve energy levels.

4. **Zinc:**

   - **Role:** Essential for immune function, wound healing, and DNA synthesis. Zinc is especially important for recovering from injuries and fighting off infections.

   - **Sources:** Meat, shellfish (especially oysters), legumes, seeds, and nuts.

   - **Example:** Studies have shown that zinc supplementation can shorten the duration of the common cold and accelerate wound healing.

5. **Iron:**

   - **Role:** Critical for producing hemoglobin, the protein in red blood cells that carries oxygen to the body's tissues. Iron deficiency can lead to fatigue and impaired cognitive function.

   - **Sources:** Red meat, poultry, seafood, lentils, spinach, and fortified cereals.

   - **Example:** A diet rich in iron (e.g., lentil soup with spinach) helps prevent anemia and boosts energy levels.

Key Takeaway:

Vitamins and minerals are essential for supporting your body's healing processes. Including a variety of micronutrient-rich foods in your diet ensures that your body has the resources it needs to heal and function optimally.

Superfoods for Healing: What You Should Be Eating Regularly

Superfoods are nutrient-dense foods that provide a high concentration of vitamins, minerals, and antioxidants, which can boost health, reduce inflammation, and promote healing. Incorporating these foods into your daily meals can have a profound impact on your well-being.

Top Superfoods for Healing

1. **Leafy Greens (Spinach, Kale, Swiss Chard):**

   - **Healing Benefits:** Rich in vitamins A, C, and K, as well as iron, calcium, and antioxidants that protect against inflammation and oxidative stress.
   - **Example:** A spinach salad with walnuts and berries provides a powerful dose of antioxidants, fiber, and essential nutrients.

2. **Berries (Blueberries, Strawberries, Raspberries):**

   - **Healing Benefits:** High in antioxidants and phytochemicals, which help protect cells from damage, reduce inflammation, and support brain health.
   - **Example:** Adding a handful of blueberries to your morning yogurt provides a boost of antioxidants that can improve memory and cognitive function.

3. **Fatty Fish (Salmon, Mackerel, Sardines):**

   - **Healing Benefits:** Rich in omega-3 fatty acids, which reduce inflammation, improve heart health, and support brain function.
   - **Example:** A grilled salmon fillet provides heart-healthy omega-3s, which can reduce the risk of cardiovascular diseases.

4. **Nuts and Seeds (Almonds, Chia Seeds, Flaxseeds):**

   - **Healing Benefits:** Packed with healthy fats, fiber, and protein, nuts and seeds support heart health, brain function, and weight management.
   - **Example:** A snack of almonds or chia pudding can provide sustained energy and help reduce cholesterol levels.

5. **Turmeric (Curcumin):**

   o   **Healing Benefits:** Known for its powerful anti-inflammatory and antioxidant properties, turmeric can help reduce joint pain and support overall health.

   o   **Example:** Adding turmeric to soups or teas can help reduce inflammation in conditions like arthritis.

Key Takeaway:

Superfoods are nature's powerhouse foods, packed with essential nutrients that support healing and reduce the risk of chronic illness. By including a variety of superfoods in your daily diet, you can nourish your body and promote long-term health.

The Healing Plate Formula: Balancing Your Meals for Maximum Health Benefits

To achieve optimal health and healing, it's important to create balanced meals that provide all the macronutrients, micronutrients, and superfoods your body needs. The Healing Plate Formula offers a simple guide for building nutrient-dense meals that promote healing and well-being.

The Healing Plate Formula

1. **Fill Half Your Plate with Vegetables and Fruits:**

   - Prioritize leafy greens, colorful vegetables, and antioxidant-rich fruits. These provide fiber, vitamins, and antioxidants that support digestion, reduce inflammation, and boost immune function.

   - **Example:** A lunch plate with half leafy greens (spinach, kale) and a mix of colorful veggies (carrots, bell peppers) paired with fresh fruit (berries or an apple).

2. **Add Lean Protein:**

   - Include a source of lean protein to support muscle repair and immune function. Aim for fish, poultry, beans, or plant-based proteins.

   - **Example:** Grilled chicken breast, baked salmon, or a plant-based option like lentils or tofu.

3. **Include Whole Grains or Complex Carbohydrates:**

   - Choose whole grains like brown rice, quinoa, or whole wheat to provide long-lasting energy and fiber.

   - **Example:** A serving of quinoa or sweet potato paired with lean protein and vegetables.

4. **Incorporate Healthy Fats:**

   - Add a source of healthy fats like avocado, nuts, seeds, or olive oil. These fats help with nutrient absorption and reduce inflammation.

- o   **Example:** Drizzle olive oil over your salad, or include a small serving of avocado or a handful of almonds.

5. **Drink Water or Herbal Teas:**

    - o   Stay hydrated by drinking plenty of water or herbal teas with your meals. Avoid sugary drinks and sodas, which can spike blood sugar and contribute to inflammation.

Sample Healing Plate Example:

- **Lunch:** Grilled salmon (lean protein), quinoa (whole grain), sautéed kale (leafy greens), roasted sweet potatoes (complex carbs), and a side of mixed berries (antioxidants) with a drizzle of olive oil (healthy fat).

Key Takeaway:

The Healing Plate Formula is a simple yet powerful tool for creating balanced meals that provide your body with the essential nutrients it needs to heal and thrive. By incorporating a variety of nutrient-dense foods in the right proportions, you can support your body's healing processes and achieve optimal health.

Creating a healing diet starts with understanding the key components of nutrition. By balancing macronutrients, incorporating micronutrient-rich foods, and focusing on superfoods, you can craft meals that not only nourish your body but also promote healing and longevity. The Healing Plate Formula provides a practical guide to building meals that are both delicious and designed to support your body's natural ability to heal.

Chapter 5

Foods to Avoid: What's Harming Your Body

In the quest for healing and optimal health, it's not just about what you eat—it's also about what you avoid. Certain foods, especially those that are highly processed or laden with sugars and unhealthy fats, can hinder your body's natural healing processes. Understanding which foods to minimize or eliminate from your diet is just as crucial as knowing which ones to include.

Highly Processed Foods and the Damage They Cause

Highly processed foods are often stripped of their natural nutrients and filled with harmful additives like preservatives, artificial flavors, colors, and unhealthy fats. These foods can cause a range of health issues and can severely compromise your body's ability to heal and function properly.

1. What Are Highly Processed Foods?

Processed foods undergo multiple changes from their original state, often for the sake of convenience, extended shelf life, or taste enhancement. This category includes foods that have been heavily altered, such as:

- Packaged snacks (chips, crackers)

- Fast food (burgers, fries)

- Sugary cereals

- Canned soups and ready-made meals

- Frozen dinners

2. The Negative Effects of Processed Foods:

- **Nutrient Deficiency:** Processing removes essential vitamins and minerals, leaving foods with empty calories that offer little to no nutritional value.

    - **Example:** A bowl of instant noodles may be quick and convenient, but it provides far fewer nutrients than a bowl of homemade vegetable soup with whole grains.

- **Artificial Additives and Preservatives:** These chemicals can disrupt your gut health, trigger allergies, and even contribute to long-term diseases.

    - **Example:** Many processed meats like hot dogs and deli meats contain nitrates and nitrites, which are linked to an increased risk of cancer.

- **Increased Inflammation:** Processed foods are often loaded with refined sugars, trans fats, and sodium, which all contribute to chronic inflammation—a root cause of many diseases, including heart disease and diabetes.

Key Takeaway:

Highly processed foods are detrimental to your health because they lack essential nutrients and are filled with harmful substances. Minimizing your intake of these foods allows your body to heal more effectively and reduces the risk of chronic illness.

Refined Sugars and Their Role in Inflammation

Refined sugars are among the most harmful ingredients in modern diets. These sugars are quickly absorbed by the body, leading to spikes in blood sugar and insulin levels, which promote inflammation and hinder healing.

1. What Are Refined Sugars?

Refined sugars are highly processed and stripped of any nutritional value. They are found in many common foods and beverages, including:

- Table sugar (sucrose)

- High-fructose corn syrup (found in sodas and many processed snacks)

- Baked goods (cakes, cookies, pastries)

- Sweetened cereals and breakfast bars

2. The Dangers of Refined Sugars:

- **Promotes Inflammation:** Excess sugar consumption triggers the release of pro-inflammatory molecules called cytokines, which contribute to chronic conditions like heart disease, diabetes, and arthritis.

    - **Example:** Regularly consuming sugary drinks like sodas or sweetened coffee can lead to chronic low-grade inflammation, which exacerbates existing health problems.

- **Impaired Immune Function:** High sugar intake weakens the immune system, making it harder for your body to fight off infections and heal wounds.

    - **Example:** Studies show that consuming large amounts of sugar can reduce the immune system's ability to kill bacteria and viruses for several hours after consumption.

- **Weight Gain and Metabolic Issues:** Refined sugars contribute to weight gain, insulin resistance, and metabolic syndrome, a collection of risk factors that increase the likelihood of developing heart disease and type 2 diabetes.

- o **Example:** A diet high in sugary snacks and beverages can lead to weight gain and insulin resistance, putting extra stress on the body and hindering healing processes.

Key Takeaway:

Refined sugars are a major contributor to inflammation and disease. Reducing or eliminating these sugars from your diet can significantly improve your health, boost your immune function, and promote healing.

Harmful Fats: Why Trans Fats and Processed Oils Slow Healing

Fats are essential for good health, but not all fats are beneficial. Trans fats and certain processed oils, such as hydrogenated oils, are particularly damaging to the body. They not only slow down healing but also contribute to inflammation and chronic illness.

1. What Are Trans Fats and Processed Oils?

- **Trans Fats:** These are artificially created fats that occur when hydrogen is added to vegetable oil, making it solid at room temperature. Trans fats are found in:

    o   Margarine and shortening

    o   Fried foods (especially those from fast food restaurants)

    o   Commercially baked goods (cookies, pastries, and cakes)

- **Processed Oils:** Many processed oils, such as vegetable oils (canola, soybean, corn oil), undergo high heat and chemical treatments during production, which strips them of their natural nutrients and causes the formation of harmful compounds.

    o   **Sources:** Processed oils are often found in salad dressings, mayonnaise, and packaged snack foods.

2. The Harmful Effects of Trans Fats and Processed Oils:

- **Increased Inflammation:** Trans fats increase the levels of inflammatory markers in the body, leading to conditions like heart disease, diabetes, and arthritis.

    o   **Example:** Regular consumption of fast food items like french fries or doughnuts, which are often fried in hydrogenated oils, can increase the risk of developing cardiovascular diseases.

- **Impaired Healing:** Trans fats interfere with the body's ability to use healthy fats, which are critical for cellular repair and inflammation control.

    o   **Example:** Replacing trans fats with healthy fats, such as those found in olive oil or avocados, improves the body's ability to heal from injuries or infections.

- **Increased Risk of Heart Disease:** Trans fats raise bad cholesterol (LDL) levels and lower good cholesterol (HDL), contributing to clogged arteries and an increased risk of heart attack or stroke.

Key Takeaway:

Avoid trans fats and processed oils to support your body's healing processes. Opt for natural, unprocessed fats like olive oil, avocados, and nuts, which promote health and reduce inflammation.

Food Allergies and Sensitivities: Identifying Hidden Triggers

Food allergies and sensitivities can cause chronic inflammation, digestive issues, and a host of other symptoms that interfere with healing. Identifying and avoiding these hidden triggers can be crucial to your overall health and well-being.

1. Common Food Allergies and Sensitivities:

- **Food Allergies:** These involve the immune system and can cause severe reactions. Common allergens include:

    - Dairy

    - Eggs

    - Peanuts and tree nuts

    - Shellfish

    - Wheat (gluten)

- **Food Sensitivities:** Unlike allergies, food sensitivities don't involve an immune response but can still cause uncomfortable symptoms like bloating, gas, fatigue, and headaches. Common triggers include:

    - Gluten (found in wheat, barley, and rye)

    - Lactose (the sugar found in dairy products)

    - FODMAPs (a group of fermentable carbohydrates found in certain fruits, vegetables, and grains)

2. Symptoms of Food Allergies and Sensitivities:

- **Gastrointestinal Issues:** Bloating, gas, constipation, or diarrhea after eating certain foods.

- **Skin Reactions:** Rashes, eczema, or acne flare-ups.

- **Fatigue and Brain Fog:** Feeling unusually tired or mentally sluggish after meals.

- **Respiratory Problems:** Congestion, coughing, or difficulty breathing in response to specific foods.

3. How to Identify Food Triggers:

- **Elimination Diet:** Remove suspected trigger foods from your diet for several weeks, then gradually reintroduce them one at a time to observe any reactions.

    o **Example:** Eliminate dairy for two weeks, then reintroduce it. If symptoms like bloating or skin irritation return, you may have a sensitivity to lactose.

- **Food Sensitivity Testing:** Work with a healthcare professional to undergo food sensitivity testing, which can help pinpoint specific triggers.

    o **Example:** Testing for gluten sensitivity or celiac disease can confirm whether gluten is contributing to digestive issues.

Key Takeaway:

Identifying and eliminating food allergies and sensitivities can significantly reduce inflammation and improve your body's ability to heal. By paying attention to how certain foods affect your body, you can tailor your diet to support your health and well-being.

The foods you avoid are just as important as the foods you eat when it comes to healing your body. Highly processed foods, refined sugars, harmful fats, and food allergens can all contribute to inflammation, chronic disease, and impaired healing. By identifying and eliminating these harmful foods from your diet, you can reduce inflammation, boost your immune system, and create an environment in which your body can heal naturally and effectively.

Chapter 6

Healing Your Gut: The Key to Whole-Body Wellness

The health of your gut is critical to the overall well-being of your body. Often called the "second brain," your gut not only digests food but also impacts your immune system, mood, energy levels, and even your mental health. Maintaining a healthy gut can be transformative, enabling your body to heal from within and function at its best.

Understanding the Gut Microbiome

The gut microbiome refers to the trillions of microorganisms—bacteria, fungi, and viruses—that reside in your digestive tract. These microbes play a key role in digestion, immune function, and even mood regulation. A balanced microbiome is essential for optimal health, while an imbalance, or "dysbiosis," can lead to a range of issues, including inflammation, autoimmune diseases, and digestive disorders.

1. What Is the Gut Microbiome?

- The gut microbiome is a complex ecosystem made up of diverse microbial species.

- These microorganisms help break down food, synthesize essential vitamins, and protect the gut lining from harmful invaders.

    - **Example:** Certain bacteria in the gut produce vitamin K and B vitamins, which are vital for blood clotting and energy production.

2. The Importance of a Balanced Microbiome:

- **Digestion and Nutrient Absorption:** A healthy microbiome ensures proper digestion and absorption of nutrients.

    - **Example:** Bacteria in the gut help break down fiber into short-chain fatty acids, which fuel the cells in the colon and protect against inflammation.

- **Immune System Regulation:** Over 70% of the immune system resides in the gut, making it a critical player in defending against pathogens and preventing chronic inflammation.

    o **Example:** The gut microbiome communicates with immune cells to distinguish between harmful and harmless substances.

- **Mood and Mental Health:** The gut produces about 90% of the body's serotonin, a neurotransmitter that influences mood, appetite, and sleep.

    o **Example:** An imbalanced microbiome has been linked to depression and anxiety, demonstrating the connection between gut health and mental well-being.

Key Takeaway:

A balanced gut microbiome is essential for overall health. It influences digestion, immunity, and even mental health. Protecting and nurturing your gut bacteria is a crucial step toward healing your body.

Probiotics and Prebiotics: Foods to Feed Your Gut

To maintain a healthy gut, it's important to nourish the beneficial bacteria living in your digestive tract. Probiotics and prebiotics are key to this process, as they help create a balanced environment where good bacteria can thrive and flourish.

1. What Are Probiotics?

Probiotics are live microorganisms that, when consumed in adequate amounts, provide health benefits by restoring the balance of good bacteria in the gut. They are found in fermented foods and supplements.

Sources of Probiotics:

- **Yogurt:** Contains live cultures of beneficial bacteria such as *Lactobacillus* and *Bifidobacterium*.

- **Kefir:** A fermented dairy drink rich in a variety of probiotic strains.

- **Sauerkraut and Kimchi:** Fermented cabbage dishes that provide live probiotics and are also high in fiber.

- **Kombucha:** A fermented tea that contains live bacteria and yeast.

2. What Are Prebiotics?

Prebiotics are non-digestible fibers that act as food for the good bacteria in the gut, promoting their growth and activity. They are found naturally in certain foods and are essential for maintaining a healthy microbiome.

Sources of Prebiotics:

- **Garlic and Onions:** Both are rich in inulin, a type of prebiotic fiber that nourishes beneficial bacteria.

- **Asparagus and Artichokes:** These vegetables contain high levels of prebiotic fibers like fructooligosaccharides (FOS).

- **Bananas:** Especially when they are slightly green, bananas provide prebiotic fibers that promote gut health.

The Synergy of Probiotics and Prebiotics:

For optimal gut health, it's important to consume both probiotics and prebiotics. While probiotics introduce beneficial bacteria into the gut, prebiotics serve as fuel for these bacteria, helping them multiply and establish a healthy balance.

Key Takeaway:

Including both probiotics (beneficial bacteria) and prebiotics (food for those bacteria) in your diet supports a thriving microbiome. Incorporating fermented foods and fiber-rich plant foods can significantly improve gut health and overall well-being.

How Gut Health Impacts Your Immune System, Mood, and Energy

The gut doesn't just help with digestion—it plays a central role in regulating your immune system, affecting your mental health, and controlling your energy levels. An unhealthy gut can contribute to a weakened immune response, mood disorders, and chronic fatigue, while a healthy gut can have the opposite effect.

1. Gut Health and the Immune System:

- **Gut-Associated Lymphoid Tissue (GALT):** This tissue is responsible for producing and regulating immune cells. It ensures that the body responds appropriately to harmful pathogens while tolerating harmless substances like food and friendly bacteria.

    - **Example:** A strong gut barrier prevents harmful bacteria and toxins from entering the bloodstream, reducing the risk of infections and autoimmune diseases.

- **Inflammation Control:** The gut microbiome helps regulate the body's inflammatory responses. An unhealthy gut can lead to chronic, low-grade inflammation, contributing to conditions like arthritis, cardiovascular disease, and even cancer.

2. Gut Health and Mood:

- **The Gut-Brain Axis:** The gut communicates with the brain through the vagus nerve and other pathways, influencing mood, stress levels, and emotional health.

    - **Example:** Gut bacteria produce neurotransmitters like serotonin, which influence mood and mental clarity. An imbalance in gut bacteria has been linked to depression and anxiety.

- **Stress and the Gut:** Chronic stress can disrupt gut health by altering the composition of the microbiome and weakening the gut barrier. This creates a vicious cycle, as a disrupted gut microbiome can, in turn, increase stress and anxiety.

3. Gut Health and Energy Levels:

- **Nutrient Absorption:** A healthy gut microbiome is essential for the absorption of key nutrients, including B vitamins and iron, which are critical for maintaining energy levels.

    - **Example:** People with gut imbalances often report chronic fatigue, partly due to poor nutrient absorption and inflammation.

- **Reduced Toxins:** A well-functioning gut helps remove toxins and waste from the body, which can otherwise contribute to fatigue and sluggishness.

Key Takeaway:

A healthy gut influences everything from your immune function to your mental health and energy levels. By improving gut health, you can strengthen your immune system, boost your mood, and enhance your vitality.

Healing Leaky Gut Syndrome: Diet Strategies to Repair the Gut Lining

Leaky Gut Syndrome occurs when the lining of the gut becomes damaged, allowing harmful substances like toxins, undigested food particles, and bacteria to "leak" into the bloodstream. This can trigger an immune response and lead to widespread inflammation, contributing to autoimmune diseases, food intolerances, and other chronic conditions.

1. What Causes Leaky Gut Syndrome?

- **Diet:** A diet high in processed foods, refined sugars, and unhealthy fats can damage the gut lining and lead to leaky gut.

- **Chronic Stress:** Prolonged stress can weaken the gut barrier and promote inflammation.

- **Medications:** Overuse of non-steroidal anti-inflammatory drugs (NSAIDs) and antibiotics can disrupt gut health and contribute to leaky gut.

- **Gut Dysbiosis:** An imbalance of good and bad bacteria can weaken the gut lining, making it more permeable.

2. Symptoms of Leaky Gut:

- Digestive issues such as bloating, gas, and diarrhea

- Food sensitivities or allergies

- Skin problems like eczema and acne

- Chronic fatigue and joint pain

- Autoimmune conditions like Hashimoto's thyroiditis or rheumatoid arthritis

3. Diet Strategies for Healing Leaky Gut:

- **Eliminate Gut-Damaging Foods:** Avoid processed foods, refined sugars, gluten, dairy, and unhealthy fats, which can irritate the gut lining.

  - **Example:** Replace processed snacks with whole, nutrient-dense options like fruits, vegetables, and nuts.

- **Focus on Anti-Inflammatory Foods:** Include foods that reduce inflammation and support gut healing, such as leafy greens, fatty fish, turmeric, and ginger.

  - **Example:** Add salmon (rich in omega-3 fatty acids) and turmeric to your diet to reduce inflammation and promote healing.

- **Incorporate Gut-Healing Nutrients:** Specific nutrients help repair the gut lining and reduce permeability, including:

  - **L-glutamine:** An amino acid that plays a key role in maintaining and restoring the integrity of the gut lining.

  - **Zinc:** A mineral that supports the immune system and helps repair the intestinal lining.

  - **Bone Broth:** Rich in collagen, gelatin, and amino acids that promote gut healing.

- **Probiotics and Prebiotics:** Supporting a healthy microbiome with probiotic-rich foods and prebiotic fibers can help restore balance in the gut and heal the gut lining.

Key Takeaway:

Leaky Gut Syndrome can be managed and healed through strategic dietary changes. By eliminating harmful foods, reducing inflammation, and incorporating gut-healing nutrients, you can repair the gut lining and restore overall health.

Gut health is foundational to whole-body wellness. The gut microbiome plays a vital role in digestion, immune function, mood regulation, and energy levels. By understanding how the gut works and focusing on nourishing it with probiotics, prebiotics, and gut-healing foods, you can enhance your overall well-being. Healing the gut, especially from conditions like Leaky Gut Syndrome, requires a thoughtful, dietary approach that supports the body's natural healing processes and leads to optimal health.

Chapter 7

Hydration and Healing

Hydration is a fundamental aspect of healing and maintaining overall health. While many people focus on diet when it comes to healing, proper hydration is equally crucial. Water is essential for detoxifying the body, supporting cellular repair, and ensuring that every system in your body functions optimally. In this chapter, we'll explore the vital role of hydration in healing, the benefits of hydrating foods and herbal teas, and practical tips to optimize your water intake for better health and faster recovery.

The Importance of Water for Healing and Detoxification

Water is the most abundant substance in the body, making up around 60% of your total body weight. Every cell, tissue, and organ depends on water to function properly. In the context of healing, water plays a crucial role in detoxification, transporting nutrients, and facilitating the body's natural repair mechanisms.

1. The Role of Water in Detoxification:

- **Flushing Out Toxins:** Water helps the kidneys filter and remove waste products from the blood. Staying hydrated ensures that toxins are efficiently eliminated from the body through urine, sweat, and breath.

    - **Example:** Without adequate hydration, toxins can accumulate in the body, leading to symptoms like fatigue, headaches, and digestive issues.

- **Liver Function:** The liver, a major detoxifying organ, requires water to break down harmful substances, such as medications, environmental toxins, and metabolic byproducts. Adequate water intake supports optimal liver function, ensuring that it can effectively detoxify the body.

    - **Example:** Chronic dehydration can hinder liver function, making it harder for the body to break down and eliminate harmful chemicals.

2. Water and Cellular Repair:

- **Hydration and Cellular Regeneration:** Water is necessary for cell repair and growth. It helps transport essential nutrients, such as oxygen and amino acids, to the cells, enabling them to heal and regenerate.

    - **Example:** After an injury, staying hydrated accelerates wound healing by providing the cells with the nutrients they need for tissue repair.

- **Regulating Body Temperature:** Water helps regulate body temperature through sweating and respiration. Proper hydration ensures that your body can cool itself effectively, especially during illness or recovery from surgery, preventing complications like overheating.

3. Water's Role in Digestion and Nutrient Absorption:

- **Aiding Digestion:** Water is crucial for breaking down food in the digestive tract, allowing the body to absorb nutrients efficiently.

    - **Example:** Drinking water before meals aids in the production of digestive enzymes and prevents issues like constipation or bloating.

- **Enhancing Nutrient Transport:** Once food is digested, water helps carry nutrients to cells throughout the body. Without sufficient hydration, your body may struggle to absorb and transport the vitamins and minerals it needs for healing.

Key Takeaway:

Water is essential for detoxification, nutrient absorption, and cellular repair, all of which are critical for healing. By staying adequately hydrated, you can support your body's natural healing processes and enhance overall health.

Healing with Herbal Teas, Broths, and Hydrating Foods

While water is the most important source of hydration, there are other healing beverages and hydrating foods that can support your health. Herbal teas, broths, and water-rich fruits and vegetables provide additional nutrients and compounds that promote healing, reduce inflammation, and improve overall well-being.

1. Healing with Herbal Teas:

Herbal teas not only hydrate but also provide a wealth of therapeutic benefits. Many herbs have anti-inflammatory, antioxidant, and immune-boosting properties that complement the healing process.

Examples of Healing Herbal Teas:

- **Chamomile Tea:** Known for its anti-inflammatory and calming properties, chamomile can soothe the digestive system, promote relaxation, and help reduce stress-related inflammation.
  - **Example:** Drinking chamomile tea before bed can improve sleep quality and reduce digestive discomfort, both of which aid in healing.

- **Ginger Tea:** Ginger is a powerful anti-inflammatory and antioxidant that supports digestion, reduces nausea, and improves circulation.
  - **Example:** Ginger tea can be particularly helpful for individuals recovering from surgery or illness, as it aids digestion and reduces inflammation in the body.

- **Peppermint Tea:** Peppermint has a cooling, anti-inflammatory effect on the digestive tract and can ease symptoms like bloating, gas, and nausea.
  - **Example:** Drinking peppermint tea after meals can soothe digestive issues and improve gut health.

- **Turmeric Tea:** Turmeric contains curcumin, a potent anti-inflammatory compound that supports healing from injury and chronic disease.

- o **Example:** Turmeric tea, combined with black pepper for enhanced absorption, can reduce inflammation and promote recovery from conditions like arthritis or heart disease.

2. Healing with Broths:

Bone broths and vegetable broths are not only hydrating but also packed with nutrients that support healing, such as collagen, amino acids, and minerals like calcium, magnesium, and potassium.

Benefits of Bone Broth:

- **Rich in Collagen and Gelatin:** Bone broth contains collagen and gelatin, which are vital for maintaining the health of connective tissues, joints, and the gut lining. This makes it particularly beneficial for healing leaky gut syndrome, joint pain, and skin conditions.

  - o **Example:** Regular consumption of bone broth can help repair the gut lining and reduce inflammation in individuals with digestive issues or autoimmune diseases.

- **Amino Acids for Repair:** Bone broth contains amino acids like glutamine, proline, and glycine, which are essential for tissue repair, immune function, and detoxification.

  - o **Example:** Glutamine is crucial for gut healing, while glycine supports liver detoxification and improves sleep quality—both important for recovery.

3. Hydrating Foods for Healing:

Certain foods naturally contain high water content and provide a variety of vitamins, minerals, and antioxidants that support hydration and healing.

Examples of Hydrating Foods:

- **Cucumbers:** Containing about 95% water, cucumbers are also rich in antioxidants and anti-inflammatory compounds, which help reduce swelling and improve skin health.

- **Watermelon:** A hydrating fruit with over 90% water content, watermelon also contains lycopene, an antioxidant that protects cells from damage and supports heart health.

- **Citrus Fruits:** Oranges, grapefruits, and lemons are not only hydrating but also packed with vitamin C, which boosts the immune system and aids in collagen production for wound healing.

- **Leafy Greens:** Vegetables like spinach, kale, and lettuce are high in water and provide essential vitamins, minerals, and fiber that support digestion and overall health.

Key Takeaway:

Hydrating foods, herbal teas, and broths not only provide water but also offer additional healing compounds like antioxidants, collagen, and anti-inflammatory agents. Including these in your daily routine can enhance your body's ability to heal and recover.

Hydration Tips for Faster Recovery and Optimal Health

Staying hydrated is essential, but many people struggle with drinking enough water daily. In this section, we'll explore practical tips for optimizing your hydration, especially when you're recovering from illness or injury.

1. Drink Water Throughout the Day:

It's better to sip water consistently throughout the day rather than consuming large amounts all at once. This ensures your body remains hydrated and can efficiently use the water you provide.

Tip: Carry a reusable water bottle with you and set reminders on your phone to take a few sips every hour.

2. Start Your Day with Water:

Drinking water first thing in the morning helps rehydrate your body after several hours of sleep and jumpstarts your metabolism.

Tip: Add a slice of lemon to your morning water to boost hydration and aid digestion.

3. Monitor Urine Color:

A simple way to gauge your hydration status is by checking the color of your urine. Clear to pale yellow urine usually indicates adequate hydration, while darker yellow may suggest that you need more water.

Tip: Aim for clear or light yellow urine throughout the day as a sign that you're staying properly hydrated.

4. Include Electrolytes:

Electrolytes like sodium, potassium, and magnesium are essential for maintaining fluid balance and supporting nerve and muscle function. You may need to replenish electrolytes if you're sweating heavily due to exercise or illness.

Tip: Instead of sugary sports drinks, opt for natural electrolyte sources like coconut water, bananas, or a homemade electrolyte drink made with water, a pinch of sea salt, and a splash of lemon juice.

5. Avoid Dehydrating Beverages:

Certain drinks, like caffeinated coffee, alcohol, and sugary sodas, can actually dehydrate the body by acting as diuretics. While moderate coffee consumption may have health benefits, it's important to balance it with adequate water intake.

Tip: For every cup of coffee or alcoholic beverage you consume, drink an additional glass of water to offset dehydration.

6. Use a Water Tracker:

If you find it difficult to remember to drink water, using a hydration app or a water tracker can help you stay on top of your intake.

Tip: There are many free apps available that allow you to track your water intake and set reminders to drink water at regular intervals.

Key Takeaway:

Staying properly hydrated is one of the simplest yet most effective ways to support healing and overall health. By incorporating hydrating foods, setting water intake goals, and avoiding dehydrating beverages, you can ensure your body has the water it needs to function optimally.

Hydration is a cornerstone of healing, detoxification, and overall health. Water helps transport nutrients, flush out toxins, and facilitate cellular repair, all of which are essential for recovery. By incorporating hydrating foods, herbal teas, and broths into your daily routine, you can boost your hydration and support your body's natural healing processes. Additionally, following practical hydration tips ensures that you remain optimally hydrated, allowing your body to recover more quickly and maintain peak health.

Part 3: Healing Through Different Life Stages and Conditions

Chapter 8

Healing Foods for Common Health Issues

In this chapter, we'll explore how specific foods and dietary strategies can help manage and alleviate common health issues. By understanding how different foods can support your body in dealing with chronic inflammation, immune system challenges, digestive disorders, and joint health, you can make informed choices that enhance your overall well-being and recovery.

Managing Chronic Inflammation Through Diet

Chronic inflammation is a persistent, low-grade inflammation that can contribute to a range of health problems, including cardiovascular disease, diabetes, and autoimmune disorders. Diet plays a critical role in modulating inflammation and promoting a healthier inflammatory response.

1. Understanding Chronic Inflammation:

- **What It Is:** Chronic inflammation is a prolonged inflammatory response that can become maladaptive, causing damage to healthy tissues and organs over time.

- **Causes:** Factors such as poor diet, stress, environmental toxins, and sedentary lifestyle can contribute to chronic inflammation.

2. Anti-Inflammatory Foods:

Certain foods contain compounds that can help reduce inflammation and support overall health. Incorporating these into your diet can help manage chronic inflammation more effectively.

Examples of Anti-Inflammatory Foods:

- **Berries:** Blueberries, strawberries, and raspberries are rich in antioxidants, such as anthocyanins, that have anti-inflammatory properties.

- **Example:** Adding a handful of berries to your breakfast or snack can help reduce oxidative stress and inflammation.

- **Fatty Fish:** Salmon, mackerel, and sardines are high in omega-3 fatty acids, which have been shown to lower levels of inflammatory markers in the body.

  - **Example:** Consuming fatty fish two to three times a week can help manage inflammation and support heart health.

- **Leafy Greens:** Spinach, kale, and Swiss chard are packed with vitamins and antioxidants that can help combat inflammation.

  - **Example:** A daily green smoothie or salad can provide a concentrated dose of anti-inflammatory nutrients.

- **Turmeric:** Curcumin, the active compound in turmeric, has potent anti-inflammatory and antioxidant effects.

  - **Example:** Incorporate turmeric into your cooking or drink turmeric tea to harness its anti-inflammatory benefits.

- **Nuts and Seeds:** Walnuts, flaxseeds, and chia seeds are rich in omega-3 fatty acids and antioxidants that help reduce inflammation.

  - **Example:** Snack on a small handful of nuts or add seeds to your meals for a boost of anti-inflammatory nutrients.

3. Foods to Avoid:

Certain foods can exacerbate inflammation and should be limited or avoided.

Examples of Inflammatory Foods:

- **Refined Sugars:** High sugar intake can increase inflammation and contribute to obesity and insulin resistance.

  - **Tip:** Opt for natural sweeteners like honey or maple syrup in moderation and choose whole fruits for sweetness.

- **Trans Fats:** Found in many processed and fried foods, trans fats promote inflammation and increase the risk of heart disease.

    o **Tip:** Avoid foods with partially hydrogenated oils and choose healthier fats, like those from avocados and olive oil.

- **Processed Meats:** Sausages, bacon, and deli meats contain compounds that can increase inflammation.

    o **Tip:** Opt for lean, unprocessed meats and plant-based protein sources.

Key Takeaway:

Diet plays a pivotal role in managing chronic inflammation. By incorporating anti-inflammatory foods and avoiding those that exacerbate inflammation, you can support your body's natural healing processes and improve overall health.

Foods to Support Immune Health

A strong immune system is essential for defending against infections and illnesses. Certain foods can enhance immune function, support your body's defenses, and reduce susceptibility to disease.

1. Understanding Immune Health:

- **Components of the Immune System:** The immune system includes various cells, tissues, and organs that work together to identify and eliminate pathogens.

- **Factors Influencing Immune Health:** Diet, stress, sleep, and lifestyle choices all impact immune function.

2. Immune-Boosting Foods:

Incorporating specific foods into your diet can provide the nutrients necessary to support and enhance immune health.

Examples of Immune-Boosting Foods

- **Citrus Fruits:** Oranges, lemons, and grapefruits are high in vitamin C, which boosts the production of white blood cells and enhances immune function.
    - **Example:** Start your day with a glass of orange juice or add lemon slices to your water for a vitamin C boost.

- **Garlic:** Contains allicin, a compound with antimicrobial and immune-boosting properties.
    - **Example:** Use fresh garlic in cooking or add garlic supplements to support immune health.

- **Ginger:** Known for its anti-inflammatory and antioxidant properties, ginger can help support immune function and reduce symptoms of illness.
    - **Example:** Drink ginger tea or incorporate fresh ginger into your meals.

- **Yogurt:** Probiotics found in yogurt support gut health, which is closely linked to immune function.
    - **Example:** Choose plain, unsweetened yogurt and add fruits or nuts for a nutritious snack.

- **Red Bell Peppers:** Rich in vitamin C and beta-carotene, which support immune health and skin integrity.
    - **Example:** Add red bell peppers to salads, stir-fries, or as a crunchy snack with hummus.

3. Foods to Avoid for Immune Health:

Certain dietary choices can impair immune function and should be limited to support overall immune health.

Examples of Immune-Compromising Foods:

- **High-Sugar Foods:** Excess sugar can suppress the immune system and increase inflammation.

    o   **Tip:** Reduce intake of sugary snacks and beverages, and choose natural sweeteners in moderation.

- **Excessive Alcohol:** Alcohol can impair the immune system and disrupt gut health.

    o   **Tip:** Limit alcohol consumption and stay hydrated with water or herbal teas.

Key Takeaway:

Supporting immune health through diet involves consuming nutrient-dense foods that boost immune function and avoiding those that can impair it. Incorporating immune-boosting foods can enhance your body's ability to fight off illness and maintain overall health.

Healing Foods for Digestive Disorders (IBS, Acid Reflux, etc.)

Digestive disorders, such as Irritable Bowel Syndrome (IBS) and acid reflux, can significantly impact quality of life. Diet plays a key role in managing symptoms and promoting digestive health.

1. Understanding Digestive Disorders:

- **IBS:** A common condition characterized by symptoms such as abdominal pain, bloating, and changes in bowel habits. Triggers can include certain foods, stress, and hormonal changes.

- **Acid Reflux:** Occurs when stomach acid flows back into the esophagus, causing symptoms like heartburn and regurgitation. It can be triggered by certain foods, overeating, and lying down after meals.

2. Foods to Relieve IBS Symptoms:

- **Low-FODMAP Foods:** The Low-FODMAP diet can help identify and eliminate foods that trigger IBS symptoms. FODMAPs are certain types of carbohydrates that can cause digestive distress.

  - **Examples:** Carrots, spinach, strawberries, and gluten-free grains are generally well-tolerated.

- **Fiber-Rich Foods:** Soluble fiber can help manage IBS symptoms by promoting regular bowel movements and reducing diarrhea.

  - **Example:** Oats, chia seeds, and bananas are good sources of soluble fiber.

3. Foods to Relieve Acid Reflux:

- **Alkaline Foods:** Foods with a higher pH level can help neutralize stomach acid and reduce symptoms of acid reflux.

  - **Examples:** Bananas, melons, and green leafy vegetables.

- **Lean Proteins:** Opt for lean sources of protein that are less likely to exacerbate acid reflux.

- o   **Examples:** Chicken breast, turkey, and tofu.

4. Foods to Avoid for Digestive Disorders:

Certain foods can aggravate IBS or acid reflux symptoms and should be minimized or avoided.

Examples of Problematic Foods:

- **High-FODMAP Foods:** Such as garlic, onions, and certain beans, which can trigger IBS symptoms.

  - o   **Tip:** Consider working with a dietitian to identify and avoid specific FODMAP triggers.

- **Spicy Foods:** Can exacerbate acid reflux symptoms and cause irritation.

  - o   **Tip:** Use mild herbs and spices for flavor instead of hot peppers or chili.

- **Caffeinated and Carbonated Beverages:** Can increase stomach acid production and exacerbate acid reflux.

  - o   **Tip:** Opt for herbal teas and still water to stay hydrated without irritating the digestive system.

Key Takeaway:

Managing digestive disorders through diet involves understanding and avoiding triggers, as well as incorporating foods that support digestive health. By focusing on healing foods and avoiding problematic ones, you can alleviate symptoms and improve overall digestive function.

Supporting Joint Health with Anti-inflammatory Foods

Joint health is crucial for maintaining mobility and quality of life, especially as you age. Inflammation in the joints can contribute to pain and conditions like osteoarthritis. Diet plays a significant role in supporting joint health and reducing inflammation.

1. Understanding Joint Health:

- **Joint Inflammation:** Conditions such as osteoarthritis and rheumatoid arthritis involve inflammation in the joints, leading to pain, stiffness, and decreased mobility.

- **Diet's Role:** Anti-inflammatory foods can help reduce joint pain and support overall joint health.

2. Anti-Inflammatory Foods for Joint Health:

- **Omega-3 Fatty Acids:** Found in fatty fish and flaxseeds, omega-3s help reduce inflammation and support joint health.

    - **Example:** Include salmon, walnuts, or flaxseed oil in your diet for a boost of omega-3s.

- **Turmeric and Ginger:** Both have strong anti-inflammatory properties that can help alleviate joint pain and stiffness.

    - **Example:** Use turmeric and ginger in cooking or take them as supplements to benefit from their anti-inflammatory effects.

- **Leafy Greens and Cruciferous Vegetables:** Spinach, kale, broccoli, and Brussels sprouts provide vitamins and antioxidants that help reduce inflammation.

    - **Example:** Include a variety of these vegetables in your daily meals to support joint health.

- **Berries:** Rich in antioxidants, berries can help reduce oxidative stress and inflammation.

    - **Example:** Add blueberries or strawberries to your breakfast or snack on them for an anti-inflammatory boost.

3. Foods to Avoid for Joint Health:

Certain foods can exacerbate inflammation and joint pain, and should be limited or avoided.

Examples of Inflammatory Foods:

- **Sugary Foods and Beverages:** High sugar intake can increase inflammation and exacerbate joint pain.

    - **Tip:** Limit consumption of sugary snacks and drinks, and choose whole fruits for sweetness.

- **Refined Carbohydrates:** White bread, pastries, and other refined carbs can contribute to inflammation.

    - **Tip:** Opt for whole grains and complex carbohydrates like quinoa and brown rice.

- **Saturated and Trans Fats:** Found in many processed and fried foods, these fats can promote inflammation.

    - **Tip:** Replace unhealthy fats with healthy fats from sources like avocados, nuts, and olive oil.

Key Takeaway:

Supporting joint health through diet involves focusing on anti-inflammatory foods and avoiding those that can increase inflammation. By incorporating beneficial foods and limiting inflammatory ones, you can reduce joint pain and improve overall mobility and health.

Healing foods play a critical role in managing and alleviating various health issues, from chronic inflammation and immune system support to digestive disorders and joint health. By incorporating nutrient-dense, anti-inflammatory foods and avoiding those that exacerbate symptoms, you can enhance your body's ability to heal and maintain overall well-being. Understanding how diet impacts these common health issues empowers you to make informed choices that promote better health and recovery.

Chapter 9

Special Diets for Healing

Special diets can offer targeted benefits for healing and overall health. By focusing on specific dietary patterns, such as the Mediterranean diet, anti-inflammatory diet, plant-based diets, and intermittent fasting, you can harness their unique healing properties to address various health concerns and promote wellness. In this chapter, we'll delve into each of these diets, exploring their principles, benefits, and how they can be implemented effectively for healing.

Healing with the Mediterranean Diet

The Mediterranean diet is celebrated for its heart-healthy benefits and its potential to promote overall wellness. Rooted in the traditional eating patterns of countries bordering the Mediterranean Sea, this diet emphasizes fresh, whole foods and healthy fats.

1. Principles of the Mediterranean Diet:

- **Focus on Whole Foods:** Emphasizes fruits, vegetables, whole grains, legumes, nuts, and seeds.

- **Healthy Fats:** Incorporates olive oil as the primary source of fat, along with nuts and seeds.

- **Lean Proteins:** Includes fish and seafood as primary protein sources, with moderate consumption of poultry, dairy, and eggs.

- **Limited Red Meat:** Red meat is consumed sparingly, often on a weekly or monthly basis.

- **Herbs and Spices:** Uses herbs and spices to flavor food instead of salt, which adds a range of beneficial compounds.

2. Health Benefits:

- **Heart Health:** The Mediterranean diet is associated with reduced risk of heart disease due to its emphasis on healthy fats and antioxidant-rich foods.

    - **Example:** Regular consumption of olive oil and fatty fish can lower LDL cholesterol levels and reduce inflammation.

- **Weight Management:** High fiber content from fruits, vegetables, and whole grains promotes satiety and helps with weight management.

    - **Example:** A diet rich in fiber helps control appetite and prevent overeating.

- **Reduced Inflammation:** The diet's focus on anti-inflammatory foods, like berries, nuts, and fish, can help reduce chronic inflammation.

    - **Example:** Including a variety of colorful fruits and vegetables in your diet provides antioxidants that combat inflammation.

3. Implementing the Mediterranean Diet:

- **Daily Meals:** Focus on incorporating a variety of fruits, vegetables, whole grains, and healthy fats into daily meals.

    - **Example:** Start with a breakfast of Greek yogurt topped with berries and nuts, enjoy a lunch of quinoa salad with mixed vegetables, and opt for grilled fish with a side of steamed greens for dinner.

- **Cooking Tips:** Use olive oil for cooking and seasoning, and incorporate herbs like basil, oregano, and rosemary for added flavor and health benefits.

    - **Example:** Prepare roasted vegetables with olive oil and rosemary for a nutritious side dish.

Key Takeaway:

The Mediterranean diet provides a comprehensive approach to healing and wellness, offering benefits for heart health, weight management, and inflammation reduction. By focusing on whole foods, healthy fats, and lean proteins, you can support overall health and promote a balanced, healing lifestyle.

The Anti-Inflammatory Diet Explained

The anti-inflammatory diet focuses on reducing chronic inflammation through food choices. Chronic inflammation is linked to various health issues, including heart disease, arthritis, and autoimmune disorders.

1. Core Principles of the Anti-Inflammatory Diet:

- **Emphasize Whole Foods:** Prioritize fruits, vegetables, whole grains, and lean proteins.

- **Incorporate Anti-Inflammatory Foods:** Include foods with known anti-inflammatory properties, such as omega-3 fatty acids, antioxidants, and polyphenols.

- **Avoid Inflammatory Foods:** Limit or avoid foods that can trigger inflammation, such as refined sugars, processed meats, and trans fats.

2. Anti-Inflammatory Foods:

- **Berries:** Rich in antioxidants and vitamins that help reduce inflammation.

    - **Example:** Add blueberries or strawberries to smoothies or oatmeal for an anti-inflammatory boost.

- **Fatty Fish:** High in omega-3 fatty acids, which have potent anti-inflammatory effects.

    - **Example:** Include salmon, mackerel, or sardines in your diet several times a week.

- **Leafy Greens:** Spinach, kale, and Swiss chard are high in vitamins and antioxidants.

    - **Example:** Prepare salads or green smoothies with a variety of leafy greens.

- **Nuts and Seeds:** Provide omega-3 fatty acids and antioxidants that help reduce inflammation.

    - **Example:** Snack on a handful of walnuts or chia seeds as part of your daily routine.

3. Foods to Avoid:

- **Refined Sugars:** Can increase inflammation and contribute to chronic disease.

  - o **Tip:** Replace sugary snacks with fruit or yogurt sweetened with honey.

- **Processed Meats:** Such as bacon and sausages, which contain inflammatory compounds.

  - o **Tip:** Choose lean, unprocessed meats and plant-based protein sources.

- **Trans Fats:** Found in many processed and fried foods, promoting inflammation.

  - o **Tip:** Opt for healthy fats from sources like avocados and olive oil.

4. Implementing the Anti-Inflammatory Diet:

- **Meal Planning:** Plan meals around anti-inflammatory foods and incorporate them into your daily diet.

  - o **Example:** Prepare a quinoa salad with mixed vegetables, nuts, and a lemon-tahini dressing for a nutritious, anti-inflammatory meal.

- **Cooking Techniques:** Use cooking methods that preserve the anti-inflammatory properties of foods, such as steaming or baking.

  - o **Example:** Bake salmon with a sprinkle of turmeric and black pepper to enhance its anti-inflammatory benefits.

Key Takeaway:

The anti-inflammatory diet focuses on reducing chronic inflammation through food choices. By emphasizing anti-inflammatory foods and avoiding those that trigger inflammation, you can improve overall health and manage chronic conditions more effectively.

Plant-Based Healing: The Benefits of Vegan and Vegetarian Diets

Plant-based diets, including vegan and vegetarian options, have gained popularity for their health benefits and their role in promoting healing. These diets focus on whole, plant-based foods and can offer significant health advantages.

1. Principles of Plant-Based Diets:

- **Vegan Diet:** Excludes all animal products, including meat, dairy, and eggs. Emphasizes fruits, vegetables, grains, legumes, nuts, and seeds.

- **Vegetarian Diet:** Excludes meat but may include dairy products and eggs. Focuses on plant-based foods with optional animal-based products.

2. Health Benefits of Plant-Based Diets:

- **Heart Health:** Plant-based diets are associated with lower cholesterol levels and reduced risk of heart disease.

    - **Example:** A diet high in fruits, vegetables, and whole grains can improve cardiovascular health and reduce blood pressure.

- **Weight Management:** Plant-based diets are often lower in calories and higher in fiber, which can aid in weight management.

    - **Example:** Eating a variety of vegetables and legumes can help you feel full and satisfied while consuming fewer calories.

- **Digestive Health:** High fiber content in plant-based diets supports healthy digestion and can prevent issues like constipation.

    - **Example:** Incorporate fiber-rich foods like beans, lentils, and whole grains into your meals for better digestive health.

- **Reduced Inflammation:** Plant-based diets rich in antioxidants and phytochemicals can help reduce inflammation.

    - **Example:** Include foods like berries, leafy greens, and nuts to combat inflammation and support overall health.

3. Implementing a Plant-Based Diet:

- **Meal Planning:** Focus on a variety of plant-based foods to ensure you get a balanced intake of nutrients.

    - o **Example:** Plan meals around legumes, whole grains, and a variety of colorful vegetables to ensure nutritional balance.

- **Supplementation:** Consider supplements for nutrients that may be challenging to obtain from a plant-based diet, such as vitamin B12, vitamin D, and omega-3 fatty acids.

    - o **Example:** Use fortified plant-based milk or a B12 supplement to ensure adequate intake.

4. Potential Challenges:

- **Nutrient Deficiencies:** Ensure you get adequate amounts of protein, vitamin B12, iron, and omega-3 fatty acids.

    - o **Tip:** Incorporate a range of plant-based protein sources, such as tofu, tempeh, and legumes, and consider fortified foods or supplements as needed.

- **Planning Balanced Meals:** It's important to plan meals carefully to avoid nutrient deficiencies and ensure a well-rounded diet.

    - o **Tip:** Work with a nutritionist to develop a meal plan that meets your nutritional needs while adhering to a plant-based diet.

Key Takeaway:

Plant-based diets offer numerous health benefits, including improved heart health, weight management, and reduced inflammation. By focusing on a variety of plant-based foods and addressing potential nutrient deficiencies, you can support healing and overall wellness through a vegan or vegetarian diet.

The Role of Intermittent Fasting in Healing

Intermittent fasting (IF) involves cycling between periods of eating and fasting. This approach has gained attention for its potential health benefits, including improved metabolic health and enhanced cellular repair processes.

1. Principles of Intermittent Fasting:

- **Fasting Windows:** Intermittent fasting typically involves restricting eating to a specific time window each day or alternating between fasting and eating days.

    - **Example:** The 16/8 method involves fasting for 16 hours and eating within an 8-hour window each day.

- **Types of Intermittent Fasting:** Common methods include:

    - **Time-Restricted Eating:** Eating within a specific time window each day, such as 12-8 PM.

    - **Alternate-Day Fasting:** Fasting every other day or significantly reducing calorie intake on fasting days.

    - **5:2 Diet:** Eating normally for five days and restricting calories to about 500-600 on two non-consecutive days.

2. Health Benefits of Intermittent Fasting:

- **Weight Loss:** Intermittent fasting can help with weight management by reducing overall calorie intake and increasing fat oxidation.

    - **Example:** The fasting periods can lead to reduced caloric intake and improved fat metabolism.

- **Improved Metabolic Health:** IF can enhance insulin sensitivity and support healthy blood sugar levels.

    - **Example:** Periods of fasting can help regulate blood sugar levels and reduce the risk of type 2 diabetes.

- **Cellular Repair and Longevity:** Fasting triggers autophagy, a process where cells remove damaged components, which can contribute to longevity and reduced risk of chronic diseases.

  - o **Example:** Extended fasting periods can enhance cellular repair mechanisms and support overall health.

3. Implementing Intermittent Fasting:

- **Choosing a Method:** Select an intermittent fasting method that fits your lifestyle and health goals.

  - o **Example:** Start with a 12/12 fasting schedule and gradually increase to a 16/8 schedule if desired.

- **Hydration:** Drink plenty of water during fasting periods to stay hydrated.

  - o **Tip:** Herbal teas and black coffee are generally acceptable during fasting hours and can help manage hunger.

- **Balanced Meals:** Focus on nutrient-dense foods during eating periods to ensure you meet your nutritional needs.

  - o **Example:** Include a mix of protein, healthy fats, and fiber-rich carbohydrates in your meals to support overall health.

4. Potential Challenges:

- **Initial Adjustment:** Some people may experience hunger, irritability, or fatigue when starting intermittent fasting.

  - o **Tip:** Gradually adjust to fasting periods and ensure adequate hydration and balanced meals to ease the transition.

- **Nutrient Intake:** Ensure you consume a balanced diet to avoid nutrient deficiencies during eating periods.

  - o **Tip:** Plan meals carefully to include a variety of nutrients and avoid processed foods.

Key Takeaway:

Intermittent fasting offers potential health benefits, including weight loss, improved metabolic health, and enhanced cellular repair. By selecting an appropriate fasting method, staying hydrated, and focusing on balanced nutrition during eating periods, you can harness the benefits of intermittent fasting for overall healing and wellness.

Special diets can provide targeted healing benefits, addressing various health concerns and promoting overall wellness. Whether you choose the Mediterranean diet, an anti-inflammatory diet, a plant-based approach, or intermittent fasting, understanding the principles and benefits of each can help you make informed dietary choices that support your healing journey and enhance your quality of life.

Chapter 10:

Eating to Heal During Different Life Stages

Our nutritional needs and the role of food in healing can vary greatly throughout different stages of life. Understanding how to tailor your diet to support health and healing during childhood, pregnancy, menopause, aging, and an active lifestyle can enhance overall well-being and resilience. In this chapter, we'll explore dietary strategies and healing foods for each of these key life stages.

Nutritional Needs for Healing in Children and Adolescents

Proper nutrition during childhood and adolescence is crucial for growth, development, and overall health. This stage of life requires a focus on foods that support physical and cognitive development, as well as healing and immunity.

1. Key Nutritional Needs:

- **Protein:** Essential for growth, tissue repair, and muscle development.

    - **Example:** Include sources like lean meats, fish, eggs, beans, and dairy products.

- **Calcium and Vitamin D:** Important for bone development and health.

    - **Example:** Provide calcium-rich foods like milk, yogurt, and leafy greens, and ensure adequate vitamin D through fortified foods or sunlight exposure.

- **Iron:** Necessary for cognitive development and to prevent anemia.

    - **Example:** Include iron-rich foods such as lean meats, fortified cereals, and legumes, and pair with vitamin C-rich foods to enhance absorption.

- **Omega-3 Fatty Acids:** Support brain development and cognitive function.

    - **Example:** Offer fatty fish like salmon or plant-based sources like flaxseeds and walnuts.

2. Healing Foods for Children and Adolescents:

- **Fruits and Vegetables:** Rich in vitamins, minerals, and antioxidants that support overall health.

    o **Example:** Encourage a variety of colorful fruits and vegetables in daily meals and snacks.

- **Whole Grains:** Provide essential nutrients and fiber for digestive health.

    o **Example:** Opt for whole grain cereals, bread, and brown rice instead of refined grains.

- **Healthy Fats:** Support brain development and overall health.

    o **Example:** Include sources like avocados, nuts, and olive oil in meals.

3. Implementing a Healing Diet:

- **Balanced Meals:** Ensure each meal includes a mix of protein, healthy fats, and complex carbohydrates.

    o **Example:** A balanced breakfast might include scrambled eggs, whole grain toast, and a side of fruit.

- **Snacks:** Provide nutrient-dense snacks to support energy levels and growth.

    o **Example:** Offer snacks like yogurt with fruit, hummus with vegetable sticks, or a handful of nuts.

Key Takeaway:

Supporting the health and healing of children and adolescents requires a focus on balanced nutrition that includes protein, calcium, iron, omega-3 fatty acids, and a variety of fruits, vegetables, and whole grains. By providing these essential nutrients, you can support optimal growth, development, and overall well-being during these formative years.

Healing Foods for Women: Pregnancy, Menopause, and Beyond

Women's nutritional needs change significantly throughout life, particularly during pregnancy, menopause, and beyond. Tailoring the diet to meet these changing needs can support overall health and healing.

1. Nutritional Needs During Pregnancy:

- **Folic Acid:** Essential for fetal development and to prevent neural tube defects.

  - **Example:** Include folate-rich foods such as leafy greens, fortified cereals, and legumes.

- **Iron and Calcium:** Important for both maternal health and fetal development.

  - **Example:** Provide iron-rich foods like lean meats and legumes, and calcium-rich foods like dairy products or fortified plant-based alternatives.

- **Omega-3 Fatty Acids:** Support fetal brain and eye development.

  - **Example:** Include fatty fish like salmon or flaxseed oil.

2. Nutritional Needs During Menopause:

- **Phytoestrogens:** Plant compounds that may help balance hormones and reduce menopause symptoms.

  - **Example:** Include soy products like tofu and edamame, and flaxseeds.

- **Calcium and Vitamin D:** To support bone health, which can be impacted by menopause.

  - **Example:** Incorporate calcium-rich foods and ensure adequate vitamin D through sunlight exposure or supplements.

- **Antioxidants:** Help combat oxidative stress and support overall health.

  - **Example:** Eat a variety of colorful fruits and vegetables.

3. Nutritional Needs Beyond Menopause:

- **Healthy Fats:** Support cardiovascular health and cognitive function.

- o **Example:** Include avocados, nuts, and olive oil in your diet.

- **Fiber:** Supports digestive health and helps maintain a healthy weight.

  - o **Example:** Focus on whole grains, fruits, vegetables, and legumes.

4. Implementing a Healing Diet:

- **Pregnancy:** Focus on balanced meals with a variety of nutrients, and stay hydrated.

  - o **Example:** A pregnancy-friendly meal might include a quinoa salad with mixed vegetables and grilled chicken.

- **Menopause and Beyond:** Emphasize foods that support bone health, hormone balance, and overall well-being.

  - o **Example:** A menopause-friendly meal might include a tofu stir-fry with broccoli and a side of quinoa.

Key Takeaway:

Tailoring nutrition to the specific needs of women during pregnancy, menopause, and beyond involves focusing on essential nutrients such as folic acid, iron, calcium, and healthy fats. By addressing these needs with a balanced diet, women can support overall health and healing throughout different life stages.

Foods for Longevity and Aging Gracefully

As we age, our nutritional needs may shift to support health, mobility, and vitality. A diet that promotes longevity and aging gracefully focuses on maintaining overall health and preventing age-related diseases.

1. Key Nutritional Needs for Aging:

- **Antioxidants:** Help combat oxidative stress and reduce the risk of chronic diseases.

    - **Example:** Include a variety of colorful fruits and vegetables, such as berries, spinach, and bell peppers.

- **Protein:** Supports muscle mass and strength, which can decline with age.

    - **Example:** Include sources like lean meats, fish, beans, and legumes.

- **Healthy Fats:** Support brain health and cardiovascular health.

    - **Example:** Opt for sources like olive oil, nuts, and fatty fish.

- **Fiber:** Promotes digestive health and helps manage weight.

    - **Example:** Focus on whole grains, fruits, and vegetables.

2. Healing Foods for Longevity:

- **Berries:** High in antioxidants and vitamins that support brain and heart health.

    - **Example:** Add blueberries or strawberries to breakfast cereals or smoothies.

- **Nuts and Seeds:** Provide healthy fats and essential nutrients.

    - **Example:** Snack on almonds or chia seeds, or add them to salads.

- **Leafy Greens:** Rich in vitamins, minerals, and antioxidants.

    - **Example:** Incorporate spinach, kale, or Swiss chard into your meals.

- **Legumes:** Provide protein and fiber for overall health.

    - **Example:** Include beans, lentils, and chickpeas in soups, salads, or stews.

3. Implementing a Longevity-Focused Diet:

- **Balanced Meals:** Ensure meals are rich in antioxidants, fiber, and healthy fats.

  - o **Example:** A meal for aging gracefully might include a salad with mixed greens, nuts, grilled chicken, and a side of quinoa.

- **Hydration:** Maintain adequate hydration to support overall health.

  - o **Tip:** Drink water throughout the day and include hydrating foods like cucumbers and watermelon.

Key Takeaway:

Aging gracefully involves focusing on a diet rich in antioxidants, healthy fats, and fiber to support overall health and longevity. By incorporating healing foods and maintaining balanced nutrition, you can enhance vitality and reduce the risk of age-related diseases.

Healing Foods for Athletes and Active Individuals

For athletes and active individuals, nutrition plays a crucial role in performance, recovery, and overall health. A diet tailored to the needs of an active lifestyle can enhance energy levels, support muscle repair, and optimize performance.

1. Key Nutritional Needs for Athletes:

- **Carbohydrates:** Provide energy for high-intensity exercise and endurance.

    - **Example:** Include whole grains, fruits, and vegetables in your diet.

- **Protein:** Supports muscle repair and recovery.

    - **Example:** Incorporate sources like lean meats, fish, eggs, and plant-based proteins.

- **Hydration:** Essential for maintaining performance and recovery.

    - **Example:** Drink plenty of water and consider electrolyte-rich beverages during intense exercise.

- **Healthy Fats:** Support sustained energy and overall health.

    - **Example:** Include avocados, nuts, and olive oil.

2. Healing Foods for Active Individuals:

- **Bananas:** Provide quick energy and potassium, which helps prevent muscle cramps.

    - **Example:** Eat a banana before or after workouts for an energy boost.

- **Greek Yogurt:** High in protein and probiotics for muscle recovery and digestive health.

    - **Example:** Have Greek yogurt with fruit and nuts as a post-workout snack.

- **Sweet Potatoes:** Rich in carbohydrates and antioxidants for energy and recovery.

    - **Example:** Enjoy baked sweet potatoes as a side dish or in a salad.

- **Chia Seeds:** High in omega-3 fatty acids, protein, and fiber for recovery and overall health.

- o **Example:** Add chia seeds to smoothies, yogurt, or oatmeal.

3. Implementing a Diet for Active Lifestyle:

- **Pre-Workout:** Focus on carbohydrates and some protein to fuel exercise.

  - o **Example:** Eat a small meal with whole grains, fruit, and lean protein 1-2 hours before working out.

- **Post-Workout:** Emphasize protein and carbohydrates to aid recovery.

  - o **Example:** Consume a meal or snack with protein and carbs, like a smoothie with protein powder, fruit, and spinach.

Key Takeaway:

For athletes and active individuals, a diet rich in carbohydrates, protein, and healthy fats is essential for energy, performance, and recovery. By incorporating healing foods and focusing on balanced nutrition, you can enhance your athletic performance and support overall health.

Eating to heal during different life stages involves tailoring your diet to meet specific nutritional needs and support overall health. From childhood and adolescence through pregnancy, menopause, aging, and an active lifestyle, understanding the role of nutrition in healing can help you make informed dietary choices and enhance well-being throughout your life. By focusing on the right nutrients and healing foods, you can support your body's needs and promote optimal health and longevity.

Part 4: Putting Healing into Practice

Chapter 11

Meal Planning for Healing

Effective meal planning is a cornerstone of a healing diet. It ensures that you consistently make healthful choices and can help you manage time, reduce stress, and support overall well-being. In this chapter, we'll provide a comprehensive guide on how to create a healing meal plan, including a sample 7-day meal plan and tips for batch cooking to make healthy eating easier and more convenient.

How to Create a Healing Meal Plan: Step-by-Step Guide

Creating a healing meal plan involves thoughtful preparation and a strategic approach to ensure that each meal supports your health and healing goals. Here's a step-by-step guide to help you create an effective and balanced meal plan:

1. Assess Your Nutritional Needs:

- **Determine Your Goals:** Identify your health goals, such as reducing inflammation, managing weight, or supporting digestive health.

    - **Example:** If you aim to reduce inflammation, focus on including anti-inflammatory foods like leafy greens, fatty fish, and berries.

- **Identify Key Nutrients:** Based on your goals, identify the essential nutrients you need, such as omega-3 fatty acids, fiber, or antioxidants.

    - **Example:** If your goal is to support digestive health, prioritize high-fiber foods like whole grains, legumes, and vegetables.

2. Plan Balanced Meals:

- **Incorporate Macronutrients:** Ensure each meal includes a balance of proteins, healthy fats, and complex carbohydrates.

- o **Example:** A balanced lunch might consist of grilled chicken (protein), quinoa (complex carbohydrate), and a side of avocado (healthy fat).
- **Include Micronutrients:** Focus on incorporating a variety of fruits and vegetables to meet your vitamin and mineral needs.
  - o **Example:** Add a colorful salad with bell peppers, tomatoes, and spinach to your dinner for a range of vitamins and minerals.

3. Create a Weekly Menu:

- **Choose Your Meals:** Select recipes or meal ideas for each day of the week, ensuring that they align with your healing goals and nutritional needs.
  - o **Example:** Plan for a hearty vegetable soup with beans for one dinner and a salmon and roasted vegetable dish for another.
- **Include Variety:** Aim for a diverse range of foods to ensure you get a wide spectrum of nutrients and prevent meal fatigue.
  - o **Example:** Rotate between different types of vegetables and proteins throughout the week.

4. Prepare a Shopping List:

- **List Ingredients:** Based on your meal plan, create a shopping list that includes all the ingredients you need for the week.
  - o **Example:** If you're making a variety of salads, list all necessary vegetables, greens, nuts, and dressings.
- **Organize by Category:** Group items by category (produce, dairy, grains, etc.) to make shopping more efficient.
  - o **Example:** Group fresh produce items together and list pantry staples separately.

5. Prepare and Store Meals:

- **Batch Cook:** Prepare larger quantities of meals or components that can be used throughout the week.

    - **Example:** Cook a large batch of quinoa or brown rice that can be used in multiple meals.

- **Store Properly:** Use airtight containers to store cooked meals and ingredients to keep them fresh.

    - **Example:** Store soups and stews in individual portions in the refrigerator or freezer for easy access.

6. Adjust as Needed:

- **Monitor and Adapt:** Pay attention to how your meal plan is working and make adjustments based on your feedback and changing needs.

    - **Example:** If you find you're consistently hungry between meals, increase the portion sizes of your snacks or add more protein to your meals.

Key Takeaway:

Creating a healing meal plan involves assessing your nutritional needs, planning balanced meals, and preparing a shopping list and meals in advance. By following a structured approach, you can ensure that your diet supports your health goals and makes healthy eating more manageable.

Sample 7-Day Healing Meal Plan

Below is a sample 7-day healing meal plan designed to support overall health and well-being. This plan includes a variety of nutrient-dense foods and balanced meals for each day.

Day 1:

- **Breakfast:** Overnight oats with chia seeds, almond milk, and fresh berries.
- **Lunch:** Quinoa salad with mixed greens, cherry tomatoes, cucumber, chickpeas, and a lemon-tahini dressing.
- **Dinner:** Baked salmon with a side of steamed broccoli and sweet potato wedges.
- **Snack:** Apple slices with almond butter.

Day 2:

- **Breakfast:** Greek yogurt with a handful of walnuts and sliced banana.
- **Lunch:** Lentil soup with a side of mixed green salad.
- **Dinner:** Stir-fried tofu with bell peppers, broccoli, and brown rice.
- **Snack:** Carrot sticks with hummus.

Day 3:

- **Breakfast:** Smoothie with spinach, banana, almond milk, and a scoop of protein powder.
- **Lunch:** Turkey and avocado wrap with whole-grain tortilla and a side of mixed fruit.
- **Dinner:** Stuffed bell peppers with quinoa, black beans, corn, and a sprinkle of cheese.
- **Snack:** A small handful of mixed nuts.

Day 4:

- **Breakfast:** Scrambled eggs with spinach and tomatoes, served with whole-grain toast.

- **Lunch:** Chickpea and avocado salad with a lemon vinaigrette.

- **Dinner:** Baked chicken breast with roasted Brussels sprouts and a quinoa pilaf.

- **Snack:** Greek yogurt with a drizzle of honey.

Day 5:

- **Breakfast:** Chia pudding made with coconut milk and topped with fresh mango.

- **Lunch:** Grilled vegetable and hummus wrap with a side of mixed greens.

- **Dinner:** Fish tacos with cabbage slaw and a side of black bean salad.

- **Snack:** Sliced cucumber with a sprinkle of sea salt.

Day 6:

- **Breakfast:** Whole-grain pancakes topped with fresh blueberries and a dollop of Greek yogurt.

- **Lunch:** Spinach and lentil salad with a balsamic vinaigrette.

- **Dinner:** Stuffed sweet potatoes with black beans, corn, and avocado.

- **Snack:** A small bowl of mixed berries.

Day 7:

- **Breakfast:** Smoothie bowl with mixed berries, spinach, almond milk, and granola.

- **Lunch:** Roasted chicken and vegetable bowl with brown rice and a side of green beans.

- **Dinner:** Vegetable curry with chickpeas served over cauliflower rice.

- **Snack:** An orange and a handful of pumpkin seeds.

Key Takeaway:

This sample 7-day healing meal plan provides a variety of balanced, nutrient-dense meals that support overall health. By incorporating a range of fruits, vegetables, whole grains, and lean proteins, you can meet your nutritional needs and support your healing goals.

Batch Cooking for Health: How to Save Time in the Kitchen

Batch cooking is a practical approach to meal preparation that can save time and ensure you always have healthy meals on hand. Here's how to effectively batch cook for optimal health and convenience:

1. Plan Your Batch Cooking:

- **Select Recipes:** Choose recipes that can be made in large quantities and stored for later use.

    - **Example:** Prepare large batches of soups, stews, or grain-based salads that can be portioned out for the week.

- **Create a Schedule:** Designate a day or time each week for batch cooking to streamline the process.

    - **Example:** Set aside a few hours on Sunday to cook and prepare meals for the upcoming week.

2. Prepare Ingredients:

- **Wash and Chop:** Wash, peel, and chop vegetables and fruits in advance.

    - **Example:** Prepare a variety of chopped vegetables that can be used in multiple recipes, such as bell peppers, onions, and carrots.

- **Cook in Bulk:** Prepare large quantities of grains, legumes, and proteins.

    - **Example:** Cook a large pot of quinoa or brown rice and store it in the refrigerator for easy meal additions.

3. Store Properly:

- **Use Airtight Containers:** Store cooked meals and ingredients in airtight containers to keep them fresh.

    - **Example:** Use glass containers with tight-fitting lids for storing soups, stews, and salads.

- **Label and Date:** Label containers with the date and contents to easily keep track of what you have on hand.

  - o **Example:** Label a container of cooked chicken with the date it was prepared for easy identification.

4. Reheat and Assemble:

- **Reheat Properly:** Reheat foods to a safe temperature to ensure they are safe to eat.

  - o **Tip:** Use a microwave, stovetop, or oven to reheat meals, depending on the type of food.

- **Assemble Meals:** Combine pre-cooked ingredients to create quick and easy meals.

  - o **Example:** Mix pre-cooked grains with roasted vegetables and a protein source for a quick and balanced meal.

5. Tips for Success:

- **Choose Versatile Ingredients:** Opt for ingredients that can be used in various recipes to maximize their utility.

  - o **Example:** Cook a large batch of chicken that can be used in salads, wraps, and soups throughout the week.

- **Keep it Simple:** Focus on simple, nutritious recipes that require minimal prep and cooking time.

  - o **Example:** Prepare basic dishes like roasted vegetables and grain bowls that can be customized with different toppings and dressings.

Key Takeaway:

Batch cooking is an efficient way to manage meal preparation and ensure you have healthy, ready-to-eat options throughout the week. By planning, preparing in bulk, and storing properly, you can save time in the kitchen and support your healing goals with ease.

Meal planning for healing involves creating a structured approach to ensure you consistently make healthful choices. By following a step-by-step guide, utilizing a sample meal plan, and implementing batch cooking strategies, you can streamline your meal preparation and support your health and healing goals effectively. With thoughtful planning and preparation, maintaining a healing diet becomes a manageable and rewarding endeavor.

Chapter 12

Healing Recipes

Cooking nourishing meals is an integral part of supporting your health and healing journey. This chapter provides a collection of healing recipes designed to energize, nourish, and support your body through various meal times. Each recipe emphasizes nutrient-dense ingredients that contribute to overall well-being and healing.

Breakfasts to Heal and Energize: Smoothies, Bowls, and More

Starting your day with a nutrient-rich breakfast can set the tone for a balanced and healthful day. These breakfast ideas are packed with vitamins, minerals, and energy-boosting ingredients.

1. Green Detox Smoothie

- **Ingredients:**

    o   1 cup spinach

    o   1/2 avocado

    o   1 banana

    o   1/2 cup pineapple chunks

    o   1 cup unsweetened almond milk

    o   1 tablespoon chia seeds

- **Instructions:**

1. Place all ingredients into a blender.

2. Blend until smooth and creamy.

3. Pour into a glass and enjoy.

- **Benefits:** Spinach and avocado provide a boost of vitamins and healthy fats, while pineapple and banana add natural sweetness and digestive benefits. Chia seeds contribute omega-3 fatty acids and fiber.

2. Berry and Quinoa Breakfast Bowl

- **Ingredients:**
    - 1 cup cooked quinoa
    - 1/2 cup mixed berries (blueberries, strawberries, raspberries)
    - 1 tablespoon honey or maple syrup
    - 1/4 cup Greek yogurt
    - 1 tablespoon flaxseeds

- **Instructions:**

1. Place quinoa in a bowl.

2. Top with berries, yogurt, and a drizzle of honey or maple syrup.

3. Sprinkle with flaxseeds and serve.

- **Benefits:** Quinoa provides a complete protein source and fiber, while berries offer antioxidants. Greek yogurt adds protein and probiotics, and flaxseeds provide additional fiber and omega-3s.

3. Sweet Potato and Black Bean Breakfast Hash

- **Ingredients:**
    - 1 large sweet potato, peeled and diced
    - 1/2 cup black beans, rinsed and drained
    - 1/2 red bell pepper, diced
    - 1/4 onion, diced
    - 1 tablespoon olive oil

- o   1/2 teaspoon cumin

- o   1/4 teaspoon paprika

- o   Salt and pepper to taste

- **Instructions:**

1. Heat olive oil in a skillet over medium heat.

2. Add sweet potato and cook until tender, about 10-12 minutes.

3. Stir in bell pepper, onion, black beans, cumin, paprika, salt, and pepper.

4. Cook for another 5 minutes until heated through.

- **Benefits:** Sweet potatoes are rich in beta-carotene and fiber, black beans provide protein and iron, and the bell pepper and onion add flavor and nutrients.

Nourishing Lunches: Salads, Soups, and Wraps

Lunchtime meals that are packed with nutrients can help sustain energy levels and keep you feeling satisfied throughout the day.

1. Mediterranean Chickpea Salad

- **Ingredients:**
    - 1 can chickpeas, rinsed and drained
    - 1/2 cup cherry tomatoes, halved
    - 1/2 cucumber, diced
    - 1/4 red onion, finely chopped
    - 1/4 cup Kalamata olives, pitted and sliced
    - 1/4 cup crumbled feta cheese
    - 2 tablespoons olive oil
    - 1 tablespoon red wine vinegar
    - 1 teaspoon dried oregano
    - Salt and pepper to taste

- **Instructions:**

1. In a large bowl, combine chickpeas, tomatoes, cucumber, onion, olives, and feta cheese.

2. In a small bowl, whisk together olive oil, red wine vinegar, oregano, salt, and pepper.

3. Pour the dressing over the salad and toss to combine.

- **Benefits:** Chickpeas provide plant-based protein and fiber, while tomatoes, cucumber, and olives add vitamins and antioxidants. Feta cheese contributes calcium and flavor.

2. Creamy Butternut Squash Soup

- **Ingredients:**
    - 1 medium butternut squash, peeled and cubed
    - 1 onion, chopped
    - 2 cloves garlic, minced
    - 1 tablespoon olive oil
    - 4 cups vegetable broth
    - 1/2 cup coconut milk
    - 1/2 teaspoon ground ginger
    - 1/2 teaspoon cinnamon

- o   Salt and pepper to taste

- **Instructions:**

1. Heat olive oil in a large pot over medium heat.

2. Add onion and garlic, and sauté until translucent.

3. Add butternut squash and vegetable broth. Bring to a boil, then reduce heat and simmer until squash is tender.

4. Use an immersion blender to puree the soup until smooth.

5. Stir in coconut milk, ginger, cinnamon, salt, and pepper. Heat through.

- **Benefits:** Butternut squash is rich in vitamins A and C, while coconut milk adds creaminess and healthy fats. Ginger and cinnamon provide additional health benefits and flavor.

3. Turkey and Avocado Lettuce Wraps

- **Ingredients:**

  - o   1/2 pound ground turkey

  - o   1/4 cup diced red bell pepper

  - o   1/4 cup diced onion

  - o   1 tablespoon olive oil

  - o   1 teaspoon paprika

  - o   1/2 teaspoon garlic powder

  - o   1 avocado, sliced

  - o   Romaine lettuce leaves

- **Instructions:**

1.   Heat olive oil in a skillet over medium heat.

2.   Add ground turkey, bell pepper, and onion. Cook until turkey is browned and vegetables are tender.

3.   Stir in paprika and garlic powder. Cook for another 2 minutes.

4.   Serve turkey mixture in lettuce leaves with avocado slices.

- **Benefits:** Ground turkey provides lean protein, while avocado adds healthy fats. Using lettuce wraps instead of bread reduces carbohydrates and adds crunch.

Healing Dinners: Plant-Based, Protein-Packed, and Nutrient-Dense Meals

Dinner is an opportunity to enjoy a balanced, filling meal that supports recovery and overall health.

1. Lentil and Spinach Stuffed Bell Peppers

- **Ingredients:**

    o   4 bell peppers, tops cut off and seeds removed

    o   1 cup cooked lentils

    o   1 cup cooked quinoa

    o   1 cup spinach, chopped

    o   1/2 cup diced tomatoes

    o   1/2 teaspoon cumin

    o   1/4 teaspoon paprika

    o   Salt and pepper to taste

    o   1/4 cup shredded cheese (optional)

- **Instructions:**

1.   Preheat oven to 375°F (190°C).

2.   In a bowl, combine lentils, quinoa, spinach, tomatoes, cumin, paprika, salt, and pepper.

3.   Stuff the bell peppers with the lentil mixture and place in a baking dish.

4.   Top with cheese if using.

5.   Bake for 30-35 minutes, until peppers are tender.

- **Benefits:** Lentils and quinoa provide protein and fiber, while spinach adds iron and vitamins. Bell peppers contribute additional nutrients and antioxidants.

2. Baked Salmon with Lemon and Dill

- **Ingredients:**

    - 4 salmon fillets

    - 1 lemon, sliced

    - 2 tablespoons fresh dill, chopped

    - 1 tablespoon olive oil

    - Salt and pepper to taste

- **Instructions:**

1. Preheat oven to 400°F (200°C).

2. Place salmon fillets on a baking sheet lined with parchment paper.

3. Drizzle with olive oil, and season with salt and pepper.

4. Top with lemon slices and fresh dill.

5. Bake for 12-15 minutes, until salmon is cooked through.

- **Benefits:** Salmon is rich in omega-3 fatty acids and protein, while lemon and dill add flavor without extra calories. This meal supports heart and brain health.

3. Sweet Potato and Black Bean Chili

- **Ingredients:**

    - 1 large sweet potato, peeled and diced

    - 1 can black beans, rinsed and drained

    - 1 can diced tomatoes

    - 1 cup vegetable broth

    - 1 onion, chopped

    - 2 cloves garlic, minced

    - 1 tablespoon chili powder

- o   1 teaspoon cumin

- o   Salt and pepper to taste

- **Instructions:**

1.   In a large pot, heat olive oil over medium heat.

2.   Add onion and garlic, and sauté until translucent.

3.   Add sweet potato, black beans, tomatoes, vegetable broth, chili powder, cumin, salt, and pepper.

4.   Bring to a boil, then reduce heat and simmer until sweet potatoes are tender.

- **Benefits:** Sweet potatoes are rich in beta-carotene, while black beans provide protein and fiber. This chili is comforting and nutrient-dense.

Snack and Dessert Ideas to Support Healing

Healthy snacks and desserts can help curb cravings and provide additional nutrients to support your healing journey.

1. Almond and Date Energy Balls

- **Ingredients:**
    - 1 cup almonds
    - 1 cup pitted dates
    - 1 tablespoon cocoa powder
    - 1 tablespoon chia seeds

- **Instructions:**

1. Place almonds and dates in a food processor and pulse until finely chopped.

2. Add cocoa powder and chia seeds, and pulse until well combined.

3. Roll mixture into small balls and refrigerate.

- **Benefits:** Almonds provide healthy fats and protein, while dates offer natural sweetness and fiber. Cocoa powder adds antioxidants.

2. Baked Apple Slices with Cinnamon

- **Ingredients:**
    - 2 apples, cored and sliced
    - 1 teaspoon cinnamon
    - 1 tablespoon honey or maple syrup (optional)

- **Instructions:**

1. Preheat oven to 350°F (175°C).

2. Arrange apple slices on a baking sheet.

3.   Sprinkle with cinnamon and drizzle with honey or maple syrup if desired.

4.   Bake for 15-20 minutes, until tender.

- **Benefits:** Apples are high in fiber and vitamins, while cinnamon adds flavor and has anti-inflammatory properties.

3. Coconut Chia Pudding

- **Ingredients:**

    - 1/4 cup chia seeds

    - 1 cup coconut milk

    - 1 tablespoon maple syrup

    - 1/2 teaspoon vanilla extract

    - Fresh fruit for topping

- **Instructions:**

1.   In a bowl, mix chia seeds, coconut milk, maple syrup, and vanilla extract.

2.   Stir well and refrigerate for at least 4 hours or overnight.

3.   Top with fresh fruit before serving.

- **Benefits:** Chia seeds provide omega-3 fatty acids and fiber, while coconut milk adds healthy fats. This pudding is a great way to enjoy a creamy, nutrient-dense dessert.

Healing recipes are an essential component of a healthful diet, providing nourishment and support for your body's recovery and well-being. By incorporating a variety of nutrient-dense foods into your breakfasts, lunches, dinners, snacks, and desserts, you can enjoy flavorful and healthful meals that promote overall health and healing. Experiment with these recipes and adapt them to fit your personal preferences and dietary needs to make healing through food a delicious and sustainable part of your lifestyle.

Chapter 13

Detox and Reset: The Power of Cleansing Foods

Detoxification is a process that supports the body's natural ability to eliminate toxins and reset its systems. By focusing on cleansing foods and gentle detox practices, you can enhance your overall health and well-being. This chapter explores the concept of detoxification, provides guidelines for safely detoxifying your body with healing foods, and offers structured 3-day and 7-day cleansing programs to help you get started.

Gentle Detoxification: Using Foods to Cleanse Your System

Gentle detoxification emphasizes using natural, whole foods to support your body's detox pathways without extreme measures. This approach helps to cleanse your system while providing essential nutrients for overall health.

1. Understanding Detoxification:

- **What is Detoxification?** Detoxification is the process by which the body eliminates or neutralizes toxins through organs like the liver, kidneys, and intestines.

    o **Example:** The liver processes toxins and waste products, which are then excreted through urine or feces.

- **Importance of Detox:** Regular detoxification supports the body's ability to function optimally and can help improve energy levels, digestion, and overall health.

    o **Example:** Reducing the burden of toxins may lead to clearer skin, better digestion, and increased vitality.

2. Foods That Support Detoxification:

- **Leafy Greens:** Spinach, kale, and Swiss chard support liver function and help remove toxins from the bloodstream.

    o **Example:** Add kale to your smoothies or salads for a nutrient boost.

- **Cruciferous Vegetables:** Broccoli, Brussels sprouts, and cauliflower contain compounds that aid liver detoxification.

  - o **Example:** Steam broccoli as a side dish to enhance its detoxifying effects.

- **Citrus Fruits:** Lemons, limes, and grapefruits provide vitamin C and antioxidants that support detoxification and immune function.

  - o **Example:** Start your day with warm lemon water to stimulate digestion and detoxification.

- **Beets:** Beets help support liver function and increase bile production for toxin elimination.

  - o **Example:** Roast or juice beets for their detoxifying benefits.

- **Garlic and Ginger:** Both garlic and ginger have antioxidant properties and support liver detoxification and digestion.

  - o **Example:** Add garlic to your stir-fries and ginger to your teas.

3. Hydration and Detoxification:

- **Importance of Water:** Staying hydrated is crucial for flushing out toxins and supporting kidney function.

  - o **Example:** Aim to drink at least 8 glasses of water per day to stay hydrated and support detoxification.

- **Herbal Teas:** Teas like dandelion root, nettle, and green tea have detoxifying properties and support liver and kidney health.

  - o **Example:** Sip on a cup of dandelion tea in the morning to aid liver function.

<h1 style="text-align:center">How to Safely Detox Your Body with Healing Foods</h1>

A safe detox approach focuses on incorporating healing foods into your diet rather than extreme fasting or restrictive diets. This method supports your body's natural detoxification processes while providing essential nutrients.

1. Preparing for a Detox:

- **Consult with a Healthcare Professional:** Before starting any detox program, it's important to consult with a healthcare provider, especially if you have underlying health conditions.

    - **Example:** Talk to your doctor if you have diabetes or other chronic conditions before beginning a detox program.

- **Gradual Transition:** Begin by slowly incorporating more detoxifying foods into your diet and reducing processed and sugary foods.

    - **Example:** Start by adding a daily green smoothie or salad to your meals.

2. Detox-Friendly Foods to Include:

- **Whole Fruits and Vegetables:** Focus on consuming a variety of colorful fruits and vegetables for their antioxidant and fiber content.

    - **Example:** Include a mix of berries, apples, and leafy greens in your meals.

- **Lean Proteins:** Opt for lean sources of protein such as fish, tofu, or legumes to support muscle repair and detoxification.

    - **Example:** Have a serving of grilled salmon or a lentil-based dish.

- **Whole Grains:** Choose whole grains like quinoa, brown rice, and oats for their fiber content and ability to support digestive health.

    - **Example:** Use quinoa as a base for salads or side dishes.

3. Foods to Avoid During Detox:

- **Processed Foods:** Minimize intake of processed and sugary foods that can contribute to toxin buildup and inflammation.

    - **Example:** Avoid foods with added sugars and artificial ingredients.

- **Excessive Caffeine and Alcohol:** Limit caffeine and alcohol consumption as they can strain the liver and interfere with detoxification.

  - o **Example:** Replace your regular coffee with herbal teas and reduce alcohol intake.

4. Incorporating Detox Practices:

- **Mindful Eating:** Pay attention to your body's hunger and fullness cues and eat mindfully to support digestive health.

  - o **Example:** Practice eating slowly and savoring each bite to enhance digestion.

- **Regular Physical Activity:** Exercise helps stimulate circulation and supports the body's natural detox processes.

  - o **Example:** Engage in moderate activities like walking, yoga, or cycling.

3-Day Healing Cleanse Program

A 3-day cleanse is a short-term program designed to give your body a gentle detox boost. This program focuses on incorporating cleansing foods and simple meal plans.

Day 1:

- **Breakfast:** Green smoothie with spinach, banana, avocado, and almond milk.

- **Lunch:** Quinoa salad with mixed greens, cucumber, cherry tomatoes, and a lemon-tahini dressing.

- **Dinner:** Baked salmon with steamed broccoli and sweet potato.

- **Snack:** Fresh fruit (e.g., apple slices) or a handful of almonds.

Day 2:

- **Breakfast:** Overnight oats with chia seeds, blueberries, and a splash of almond milk.

- **Lunch:** Lentil soup with a side of mixed green salad.

- **Dinner:** Stuffed bell peppers with quinoa, black beans, corn, and a sprinkle of cheese (optional).

- **Snack:** Carrot sticks with hummus or a small bowl of mixed berries.

Day 3:

- **Breakfast:** Chia pudding with coconut milk and topped with fresh mango.

- **Lunch:** Grilled vegetable wrap with hummus in a whole-grain tortilla.

- **Dinner:** Sweet potato and black bean chili with a side of mixed greens.

- **Snack:** Greek yogurt with a drizzle of honey and a few walnuts.

Key Takeaway:

The 3-day cleanse focuses on nutrient-dense foods that support detoxification and overall health. By incorporating these meals, you can give your body a gentle reset while providing essential nutrients.

7-Day Healing Cleanse Program

A 7-day cleanse provides a more extended period for detoxification and allows for a greater variety of healing foods. This program helps you establish healthy eating patterns and supports long-term well-being.

Day 1-3:

- Follow the same meal plan as the 3-day cleanse to start your detox journey.

Day 4:

- **Breakfast:** Smoothie bowl with spinach, mixed berries, almond milk, and granola.

- **Lunch:** Mediterranean chickpea salad with a lemon vinaigrette.

- **Dinner:** Roasted chicken breast with quinoa and a side of steamed green beans.

- **Snack:** Fresh fruit or a small handful of nuts.

Day 5:

- **Breakfast:** Sweet potato hash with black beans and avocado.

- **Lunch:** Creamy butternut squash soup with a side salad.

- **Dinner:** Grilled tofu with sautéed kale and brown rice.

- **Snack:** Cucumber slices with a sprinkle of sea salt.

Day 6:

- **Breakfast:** Chia seed pudding with fresh strawberries and a drizzle of honey.

- **Lunch:** Spinach and lentil salad with balsamic vinaigrette.

- **Dinner:** Baked cod with a side of roasted Brussels sprouts and sweet potato.

- **Snack:** Greek yogurt with a handful of granola.

Day 7:

- **Breakfast:** Green detox smoothie with kale, avocado, apple, and coconut water.

- **Lunch:** Roasted vegetable and hummus wrap with a side of mixed fruit.

- **Dinner:** Stuffed zucchini boats with quinoa, tomatoes, and feta cheese.

- **Snack:** A small bowl of mixed berries or a piece of dark chocolate.

Key Takeaway:

The 7-day cleanse program provides a more extended detox period and incorporates a variety of healing foods. This approach helps to deepen the detox process while promoting lasting healthy eating habits.

Detoxification through cleansing foods can support your body's natural ability to eliminate toxins and enhance overall health. By focusing on gentle, food-based detox strategies and following structured cleanse programs, you can effectively support your body's detoxification processes. Whether you opt for a short 3-day cleanse or a more extended 7-day program, incorporating these healing foods and practices into your routine can help you feel rejuvenated and refreshed.

Chapter 14

The Healing Mindset: Combining Nutrition with Lifestyle Changes

To fully embrace the power of healing through food, it is essential to integrate nutrition with other critical aspects of lifestyle. A holistic approach that includes adequate sleep, stress management, physical activity, and mindful eating can significantly enhance your overall health and support long-term healing. This chapter explores how combining these elements with a healing diet creates a comprehensive strategy for improved well-being.

The Importance of Sleep, Stress Management, and Physical Activity

Achieving optimal health and healing requires attention to more than just nutrition. Sleep, stress management, and physical activity are vital components that influence your overall well-being.

1. The Role of Sleep in Healing:

- **Why Sleep Matters:** Quality sleep is crucial for physical and mental recovery. During sleep, the body repairs tissues, regulates hormones, and supports immune function.

    - **Example:** Growth hormone is released during deep sleep, aiding in tissue repair and muscle growth.

- **Tips for Better Sleep:**

    - **Establish a Routine:** Go to bed and wake up at the same time each day to regulate your internal clock.

        - **Example:** Aim for 7-9 hours of sleep per night, and create a relaxing bedtime routine.

    - **Create a Sleep-Friendly Environment:** Ensure your bedroom is cool, dark, and quiet.

        - **Example:** Use blackout curtains and a white noise machine if necessary.

- o **Limit Screen Time:** Avoid screens at least an hour before bed to reduce exposure to blue light, which can interfere with sleep.

2. Managing Stress for Optimal Health:

- **Impact of Stress on the Body:** Chronic stress can impair immune function, disrupt digestion, and increase the risk of chronic diseases.
  - o **Example:** Stress can lead to inflammation, which exacerbates conditions like arthritis and cardiovascular disease.

- **Stress Management Techniques:**
  - o **Mindfulness and Meditation:** Practice mindfulness meditation to reduce stress and improve emotional well-being.
    - **Example:** Spend 10-15 minutes each day practicing deep breathing or guided meditation.
  - o **Exercise:** Regular physical activity can help reduce stress and boost mood.
    - **Example:** Engage in activities like walking, yoga, or swimming to relieve stress.
  - o **Time Management:** Prioritize tasks and set realistic goals to avoid feeling overwhelmed.
    - **Example:** Use a planner to organize daily tasks and set aside time for relaxation.

3. The Benefits of Physical Activity:

- **How Exercise Supports Healing:** Regular exercise improves cardiovascular health, boosts mood, and enhances immune function.
  - o **Example:** Physical activity increases blood flow, which helps deliver nutrients and oxygen to tissues.

- **Types of Beneficial Exercise:**

  - **Aerobic Exercise:** Activities like walking, running, and cycling improve cardiovascular health.

    - **Example:** Aim for at least 150 minutes of moderate-intensity aerobic exercise per week.

  - **Strength Training:** Building muscle through resistance exercises supports metabolic health.

    - **Example:** Incorporate strength training exercises like weightlifting or bodyweight exercises twice a week.

  - **Flexibility and Balance:** Practices like yoga and stretching improve flexibility and reduce the risk of injury.

    - **Example:** Add yoga sessions or stretching routines to your weekly fitness plan.

Mindful Eating: Connecting with Your Food for Better Health

Mindful eating involves paying full attention to the experience of eating and drinking. It helps you develop a healthier relationship with food and enhances your overall well-being.

1. Principles of Mindful Eating:

- **Focus on the Present Moment:** Pay attention to the taste, texture, and aroma of your food without distractions.

    o **Example:** Eat without watching TV or using your phone, and savor each bite.

- **Listen to Your Body's Hunger Cues:** Eat when you are hungry and stop when you are satisfied, rather than eating out of habit or emotion.

    o **Example:** Use a hunger scale (1-10) to gauge your level of hunger and fullness.

- **Appreciate Your Food:** Take time to acknowledge the effort and resources that went into preparing your meal.

    o **Example:** Express gratitude for the ingredients and the nourishment they provide.

2. Benefits of Mindful Eating:

- **Improved Digestion:** Eating slowly and chewing thoroughly aids in digestion and nutrient absorption.

    o **Example:** Chew each bite 20-30 times to break down food more effectively.

- **Better Portion Control:** Mindful eating helps you recognize when you are full, which can prevent overeating.

    o **Example:** Use smaller plates and serve yourself smaller portions to avoid overeating.

- **Enhanced Enjoyment:** Mindful eating increases your enjoyment of food and helps you develop a more positive relationship with eating.

o   **Example:** Take time to enjoy the flavors and textures of each meal, making mealtime a more enjoyable experience.

Creating Long-Term Habits for Sustained Healing

Building lasting habits is essential for maintaining a healing lifestyle and achieving long-term health benefits.

1. Setting Realistic Goals:

- **Start Small:** Begin with manageable changes and gradually build on them.

    - **Example:** If you're new to exercise, start with short walks and gradually increase your activity level.

- **Track Your Progress:** Keep a journal or use an app to monitor your diet, sleep, exercise, and stress levels.

    - **Example:** Record your daily meals, sleep patterns, and exercise routines to track improvements and identify areas for adjustment.

2. Creating a Supportive Environment:

- **Surround Yourself with Support:** Engage with friends, family, or support groups who encourage your health goals.

    - **Example:** Join a cooking class or exercise group to stay motivated and share experiences.

- **Make Healthy Choices Accessible:** Stock your kitchen with nutritious foods and create a home environment that supports your healing goals.

    - **Example:** Keep fresh fruits, vegetables, and healthy snacks readily available to encourage better eating habits.

3. Embracing Flexibility and Adaptability:

- **Be Flexible:** Allow yourself to adapt your goals and strategies as needed to fit your changing needs and circumstances.

    - **Example:** If your schedule changes, find alternative ways to incorporate exercise or meal prep.

- **Practice Self-Compassion:** Acknowledge that setbacks are a natural part of the process and focus on progress rather than perfection.

  - **Example:** If you miss a workout or indulge in a less healthy meal, forgive yourself and refocus on your goals.

Integrating nutrition with lifestyle changes is crucial for achieving and maintaining optimal health. By prioritizing sleep, managing stress, engaging in regular physical activity, and practicing mindful eating, you create a comprehensive approach to healing. Building long-term habits and fostering a supportive environment further enhance your ability to sustain these positive changes. Embracing a holistic mindset and combining these elements with a nourishing diet can lead to a healthier, more balanced life.

Part 5: Sustainable Healing

Chapter 15

Navigating the Modern Food Environment

In today's fast-paced world, navigating the modern food environment can be challenging, especially when trying to maintain a healing diet. From dining out to understanding food labels and making informed choices about food sourcing, this chapter will guide you through practical strategies to ensure that you stay on track with your health goals while adapting to various eating situations.

How to Choose Healing Foods at Restaurants and Social Events.

Eating out or attending social events can present challenges, but with a bit of preparation and knowledge, you can still make choices that support your healing journey.

1. Choosing Healing Foods at Restaurants:

- **Research Ahead:** Look up the restaurant's menu online before you go. Many restaurants now offer nutritional information and ingredient lists on their websites.

  - **Example:** Choose restaurants that offer a range of fresh, whole food options or ones that cater to dietary preferences like vegetarian or gluten-free.

- **Ask Questions:** Don't hesitate to ask the server about how dishes are prepared and what ingredients are used.

  - **Example:** Inquire if a dish can be made with olive oil instead of butter or if it can be customized to include extra vegetables.

- **Focus on Whole Foods:** Opt for dishes that are rich in vegetables, lean proteins, and whole grains. Avoid heavily processed items and those with excessive added sugars or unhealthy fats.

  - **Example:** Choose a grilled chicken salad with a vinaigrette dressing over fried chicken and creamy dressings.

- **Portion Control:** Restaurant portions can be larger than necessary. Consider sharing a dish or asking for a to-go box to save half of your meal for later.

  - o **Example:** Order an appetizer as your main course or split a main dish with a dining companion.

2. Navigating Social Events:

- **Eat Before You Go:** If you're unsure of the food options at the event, have a healthy snack before you arrive to avoid arriving hungry and making less optimal choices.

  - o **Example:** Snack on a piece of fruit or a handful of nuts before the event.

- **Bring a Dish:** If it's a potluck or buffet-style event, bring a healthy dish that you know you can enjoy and share with others.

  - o **Example:** Prepare a quinoa salad with fresh vegetables or a fruit platter.

- **Practice Moderation:** If less healthy options are available, practice moderation and focus on filling your plate with the healthiest choices available.

  - o **Example:** Choose a small portion of a richer dish and balance it with a larger serving of vegetables or a salad.

Reading Labels: Decoding Ingredients and Nutritional Information

Understanding food labels is essential for making informed choices and avoiding ingredients that may hinder your healing process.

1. Understanding Nutritional Information:

- **Serving Size:** Pay attention to the serving size listed on the label to understand how the nutritional information applies to the amount you consume.

    - **Example:** A bag of chips may list the nutrition facts for a small serving, but if you eat the whole bag, you need to multiply the values accordingly.

- **Calories and Macronutrients:** Monitor the calorie content and macronutrient breakdown (fats, proteins, carbohydrates) to ensure that the product fits within your dietary goals.

    - **Example:** Look for products with a balanced macronutrient profile that aligns with your needs, such as a snack with a good mix of protein and healthy fats.

2. Decoding Ingredients:

- **Whole Food Ingredients:** Favor products with whole food ingredients and minimal processing. Ingredients should be recognizable and unprocessed.

    - **Example:** Choose oatmeal with whole oats as the first ingredient rather than products with added sugars and artificial flavors.

- **Avoiding Additives:** Be cautious of ingredients like artificial sweeteners, preservatives, and colorings, which can be detrimental to health.

    - **Example:** Avoid products with high fructose corn syrup, artificial dyes, and long lists of unrecognizable chemical names.

- **Allergen Information:** Check for potential allergens and food sensitivities, especially if you have known allergies or intolerances.

    - **Example:** Look for allergen warnings on labels if you have a sensitivity to gluten, dairy, or nuts.

3. Organic, Local, or Conventional: What's Best for Healing?

- **Organic Foods:** Organic foods are grown without synthetic pesticides, fertilizers, or genetically modified organisms (GMOs), which may offer benefits for health and sustainability.

  - **Example:** Choosing organic produce may reduce exposure to pesticide residues.

- **Local Foods:** Locally sourced foods are often fresher and may have a lower environmental impact due to reduced transportation needs. They also support local farmers and economies.

  - **Example:** Visit farmers' markets to find seasonal fruits and vegetables that are grown in your region.

- **Conventional Foods:** While conventional foods are generally safe, they may be grown with synthetic pesticides and fertilizers. Prioritize washing produce thoroughly and making informed choices based on your priorities.

  - **Example:** If buying conventional produce, use a vegetable wash or scrub to remove residues.

4. Making Informed Choices:

- **Balance and Budget:** Consider your budget and priorities when choosing between organic, local, and conventional options. Balance cost with health benefits.

  - **Example:** You might choose to buy organic for the "Dirty Dozen" produce items with higher pesticide residues while opting for conventional options for the "Clean Fifteen."

- **Environmental and Ethical Considerations:** Beyond health, consider the environmental impact and ethical practices of your food sources.

  - **Example:** Support brands and farmers that practice sustainable and ethical farming methods.

Navigating the modern food environment requires a blend of preparation, awareness, and informed decision-making. By making mindful choices at restaurants and social events, understanding food labels, and balancing your food sources, you can stay true to your healing goals while adapting to various eating situations. Embrace these strategies to maintain a healing diet and support your overall health in a complex food landscape.

Chapter 16

Overcoming Challenges in Your Healing Journey

Embarking on a healing journey through nutrition can come with various challenges. From dealing with cravings and emotional eating to managing a healing diet on a budget and staying motivated, understanding and addressing these obstacles is key to achieving long-term success. This chapter provides practical strategies and insights to help you navigate and overcome common challenges on your path to better health.

Dealing with Cravings and Emotional Eating

Cravings and emotional eating can be significant hurdles in maintaining a healing diet. Recognizing these patterns and employing strategies to address them can help you stay on track with your health goals.

1. Understanding Cravings:

- **Types of Cravings:**

    o **Physical Cravings:** Often related to nutrient deficiencies or habitual patterns.

        ▪ **Example:** A craving for chocolate might indicate a need for magnesium.

    o **Emotional Cravings:** Linked to stress, boredom, or emotional states rather than physical hunger.

        ▪ **Example:** Eating ice cream when feeling stressed or anxious.

- **Identifying Triggers:** Pay attention to what triggers your cravings. Keeping a food and mood journal can help identify patterns.

    o **Example:** If you notice that cravings often occur during stressful situations, this may indicate an emotional eating pattern.

2. Strategies to Manage Cravings:

- **Balanced Meals:** Ensure your meals are balanced with adequate protein, healthy fats, and fiber to help maintain stable blood sugar levels and reduce cravings.

  - **Example:** A meal including grilled chicken, quinoa, and a variety of vegetables can help keep you full and satisfied.

- **Healthy Substitutes:** Find healthier alternatives to satisfy cravings without derailing your diet.

  - **Example:** Swap out sugary snacks with fresh fruit or a handful of nuts.

- **Mindful Eating:** Practice mindful eating to recognize true hunger and satisfaction cues. This can help reduce the likelihood of eating out of boredom or emotional triggers.

  - **Example:** Eat slowly and savor each bite to enhance your connection with your food and reduce overeating.

3. Addressing Emotional Eating:

- **Emotional Awareness:** Recognize when you're eating in response to emotions rather than hunger. Develop alternative coping strategies for emotional stress.

  - **Example:** Practice relaxation techniques such as deep breathing or journaling instead of reaching for food.

- **Healthy Habits:** Develop healthy habits that address emotional needs and stress in non-food-related ways.

  - **Example:** Engage in activities like exercise, hobbies, or social interactions to manage stress and improve your mood.

Sticking to a Healing Diet on a Budget

Maintaining a healing diet doesn't have to be expensive. With strategic planning and smart choices, you can eat healthily while managing your budget.

1. Budget-Friendly Strategies:

- **Plan Your Meals:** Create a weekly meal plan to ensure you buy only what you need, reducing food waste and impulsive purchases.

    - **Example:** Plan meals around seasonal produce and sales to maximize your budget.

- **Buy in Bulk:** Purchase non-perishable items like grains, beans, and nuts in bulk to save money.

    - **Example:** Buy large bags of rice or dried beans and store them properly to extend their shelf life.

- **Use Coupons and Sales:** Take advantage of store coupons, sales, and loyalty programs to get discounts on healthy foods.

    - **Example:** Check weekly ads for promotions on fresh produce and lean proteins.

2. Choosing Budget-Friendly Foods:

- **Seasonal and Local Produce:** Opt for seasonal and locally grown fruits and vegetables, which are often more affordable and fresher.

    - **Example:** Purchase apples and squash in the fall, or tomatoes and zucchini in the summer.

- **Affordable Protein Sources:** Incorporate cost-effective protein sources like eggs, beans, lentils, and tofu.

    - **Example:** Prepare meals with lentils or beans, which are both nutritious and economical.

- **Frozen and Canned Options:** Use frozen fruits and vegetables or canned goods (without added sugars or salts) as budget-friendly alternatives.

    o **Example:** Keep frozen spinach and berries on hand for smoothies and soups.

3. Cooking at Home:

- **Batch Cooking:** Prepare and freeze meals in advance to save time and reduce the temptation to eat out.

    o **Example:** Cook a large batch of soup or chili and freeze individual portions for convenient, healthy meals.

- **Simple Recipes:** Focus on simple, whole-food recipes that require fewer ingredients and are cost-effective.

    o **Example:** Prepare a vegetable stir-fry with brown rice and a simple homemade sauce for a nutritious, affordable meal.

Staying Motivated: How to Keep Your Healing Diet on Track

Maintaining motivation is crucial for adhering to a healing diet and achieving your long-term health goals. Here are strategies to help you stay committed and focused on your journey.

1. Set Clear and Achievable Goals:

- **Define Your Objectives:** Set specific, measurable, achievable, relevant, and time-bound (SMART) goals to guide your progress.

    - **Example:** Aim to include at least two servings of vegetables in each meal for the next month.

- **Track Your Progress:** Keep a journal or use an app to track your meals, progress, and any changes in your health and well-being.

    - **Example:** Record your daily food intake and how you feel to identify improvements and areas needing adjustment.

2. Build a Support System:

- **Engage with Others:** Connect with friends, family, or support groups who share your health goals and can offer encouragement and accountability.

    - **Example:** Join a local or online health-focused group to share experiences and gain motivation.

- **Seek Professional Guidance:** Consult with a registered dietitian or nutritionist for personalized advice and support tailored to your needs.

    - **Example:** Schedule regular check-ins with a dietitian to review your progress and adjust your diet plan as needed.

3. Celebrate Successes:

- **Acknowledge Achievements:** Celebrate your milestones and successes, no matter how small, to stay motivated and reinforce positive behaviors.

    - **Example:** Reward yourself with a non-food-related treat, like a new book or a relaxing massage, when you reach a health goal.

- **Reflect on Your Journey:** Regularly review your progress and remind yourself of the reasons you started your healing journey.

  - o **Example:** Reflect on the positive changes you've experienced, such as increased energy levels or improved digestion.

4. Stay Flexible and Adaptable:

- **Embrace Change:** Be prepared to adapt your plan as needed and remain flexible when faced with challenges or changes in circumstances.

  - o **Example:** If you encounter a dietary setback or travel, adjust your plan to accommodate your situation while staying focused on your long-term goals.

- **Learn from Setbacks:** View setbacks as opportunities for learning and growth rather than failures. Identify what went wrong and how you can adjust your approach moving forward.

  - o **Example:** If you find yourself slipping into old eating habits, analyze the triggers and develop strategies to address them.

The Transformative Power of Food: Recap of Key Takeaways

Throughout this book, we have delved into the profound impact that food can have on your health and healing journey. Here's a summary of the crucial insights and strategies:

1. The Science of Food and Healing:

- **Natural Healing Mechanisms:** Your body has inherent capabilities to repair and restore itself. Nutrition plays a vital role in supporting these processes.

- **Food as Medicine:** Nutrient-dense foods, anti-inflammatory ingredients, and a healthy gut microbiome are central to effective healing. Phytochemicals and antioxidants act as natural healers by combating oxidative stress and inflammation.

2. Creating Your Healing Diet:

- **Healing Plate:** A balanced diet includes macronutrients (fats, carbs, proteins) and micronutrients (vitamins, minerals), with a focus on superfoods that enhance health.

- **Foods to Avoid:** Highly processed foods, refined sugars, harmful fats, and potential allergens can hinder healing. Understanding and avoiding these will support better health outcomes.

- **Healing Your Gut:** A healthy gut is crucial for overall wellness. Incorporate probiotics, prebiotics, and strategies to heal gut lining to improve immune function and digestion.

3. Healing Through Different Life Stages and Conditions:

- **Specific Diets for Health Issues:** Tailor your diet to manage chronic inflammation, support immune health, and address specific conditions like diabetes or digestive disorders.

- **Special Diets:** Explore various dietary patterns such as the Mediterranean diet, anti-inflammatory diet, plant-based eating, and intermittent fasting to find what best supports your healing.

4. Putting Healing into Practice:

- **Meal Planning:** Plan meals, create a 7-day healing meal plan, and use batch cooking to simplify healthy eating.

- **Recipes:** Enjoy a variety of healing recipes, from energizing breakfasts to nourishing lunches, dinners, and snacks.

- **Detox and Reset:** Implement gentle detoxification strategies and cleansing programs to refresh and support your body's natural healing processes.

5. Sustainable Healing:

- **Modern Food Environment:** Navigate dining out and social events, decode food labels, and choose between organic, local, and conventional foods to align with your healing goals.

- **Overcoming Challenges:** Address cravings, manage your diet on a budget, and stay motivated with practical strategies and support systems.

Your Personalized Healing Journey: Adapting What You've Learned

Each individual's path to healing is unique. Tailoring the principles and strategies outlined in this book to fit your personal needs and circumstances will maximize their effectiveness. Here's how to adapt what you've learned to create a personalized healing plan:

1. Assess Your Needs:

- **Evaluate Your Health Goals:** Reflect on your specific health goals and challenges. Are you managing a chronic condition, aiming for general wellness, or seeking to improve specific aspects of your health?

    o **Example:** If you have a condition like diabetes, focus on foods that stabilize blood sugar and avoid those that cause spikes.

- **Personalize Your Diet:** Modify the general recommendations to fit your dietary preferences, lifestyle, and any allergies or intolerances.

    o **Example:** If you're vegetarian, emphasize plant-based sources of protein and ensure you're meeting your nutrient needs.

2. Create a Flexible Plan:

- **Set Realistic Goals:** Develop a plan with achievable milestones and be flexible in adjusting it as needed based on your progress and feedback.

    o **Example:** Start by incorporating more vegetables into your meals and gradually increase other healing practices.

- **Monitor and Adjust:** Regularly review your progress, listen to your body's responses, and adjust your diet and lifestyle as needed to stay aligned with your health goals.

    o **Example:** If you notice improvements in energy levels, continue with the dietary changes and explore additional areas for enhancement.

3. Seek Support and Resources:

- **Consult Professionals:** Work with a dietitian, nutritionist, or healthcare provider to get personalized guidance and support.

- o **Example:** A nutritionist can help you design a meal plan that fits your healing needs and preferences.

- **Engage with Communities:** Join support groups or online communities that share your health interests to gain motivation, advice, and encouragement.

  - o **Example:** Participate in forums or local groups focused on healthy eating and wellness.

Next Steps: Staying on the Path to Long-Term Wellness

Maintaining long-term wellness requires ongoing commitment and adaptability. Here are steps to ensure you continue on the path to sustained health:

1. Develop Lasting Habits:

- **Integrate Healthy Practices:** Incorporate healing habits into your daily routine and make them a natural part of your lifestyle.

  - **Example:** Make meal planning, exercise, and mindfulness a regular part of your weekly schedule.

- **Continuously Learn:** Stay informed about new research, trends, and practices related to nutrition and wellness.

  - **Example:** Read reputable health blogs, attend workshops, or take online courses to stay updated.

2. Cultivate a Positive Mindset:

- **Embrace Progress:** Celebrate your achievements and remain positive about the journey, even when facing setbacks.

  - **Example:** Reflect on the benefits you've experienced and use them as motivation to continue.

- **Practice Resilience:** Be prepared to adapt and overcome obstacles, recognizing that healing is an ongoing process.

  - **Example:** If you encounter a dietary challenge, address it with a problem-solving approach and adjust your plan as needed.

3. Foster a Supportive Environment:

- **Surround Yourself with Positivity:** Build a network of supportive individuals who encourage your health goals and share your values.

  - **Example:** Engage with friends and family who support your healing journey and participate in activities that reinforce your commitment to wellness.

- **Maintain Your Focus:** Keep your health goals and reasons for pursuing a healing diet at the forefront of your mind to stay motivated.

  - **Example:** Create visual reminders or keep a journal to track your goals and progress.

The journey to healing through food is a dynamic and personal experience. By applying the knowledge and strategies from this book, you can navigate the challenges and opportunities that come your way, creating a path to lasting health and wellness. Embrace the transformative power of food, adapt what you've learned to fit your unique needs, and stay committed to your long-term goals. Your healing journey is ongoing, and with dedication and adaptability, you can achieve a vibrant and balanced life.

Appendices

The appendices of this book provide additional resources and reference materials to support your healing journey. These sections are designed to offer comprehensive information, practical tools, and further reading to help you implement and expand on the concepts discussed throughout the book.

Appendix A: Comprehensive Food Lists for Healing

This appendix provides detailed lists of foods categorized by their healing properties, making it easier to plan meals and make informed choices that support your health goals.

1. Nutrient-Dense Foods:

- **Fruits:** Blueberries, strawberries, oranges, apples, bananas, kiwi

    o **Benefits:** High in vitamins, antioxidants, and fiber

- **Vegetables:** Spinach, kale, broccoli, bell peppers, carrots, sweet potatoes

    o **Benefits:** Rich in vitamins, minerals, and phytonutrients

- **Whole Grains:** Quinoa, brown rice, oats, barley, farro

    o **Benefits:** Provide fiber, B vitamins, and minerals

- **Lean Proteins:** Chicken breast, turkey, tofu, legumes, fish (salmon, sardines)

    o **Benefits:** Support muscle repair and provide essential amino acids

2. Anti-Inflammatory Foods:

- **Spices:** Turmeric, ginger, cinnamon, garlic

    o **Benefits:** Help reduce inflammation and oxidative stress

- **Healthy Fats:** Avocados, olive oil, nuts (almonds, walnuts), seeds (chia, flax)

    o **Benefits:** Provide essential fatty acids and reduce inflammation

3. Probiotic and Prebiotic Foods:

- **Probiotics:** Yogurt, kefir, sauerkraut, kimchi, miso

    o **Benefits:** Support gut health and balance microbiome

- **Prebiotics:** Bananas, onions, garlic, leeks, asparagus

    o **Benefits:** Feed beneficial gut bacteria and improve digestion

4. Hydrating Foods:

- **Cucumbers, Watermelon, Celery, Strawberries**

    o **Benefits:** High water content to aid hydration and detoxification

Appendix B: Supplement Recommendations to Enhance Healing

While whole foods should be the primary source of nutrition, certain supplements can complement a healing diet and address specific needs. Consult with a healthcare provider before starting any new supplements.

1. Common Supplements:

- **Multivitamins:** To cover potential gaps in your diet and provide a broad range of nutrients

    - **Example:** Choose a multivitamin tailored to your age and gender.

- **Omega-3 Fatty Acids:** For reducing inflammation and supporting heart health

    - **Example:** Fish oil supplements or algae-based omega-3s.

- **Vitamin D:** To support bone health and immune function, especially in areas with limited sunlight

    - **Example:** Vitamin D3 supplements.

- **Probiotics:** To enhance gut health and balance microbiome

    - **Example:** Choose a high-quality probiotic with diverse strains.

- **Magnesium:** To support muscle function, relaxation, and overall well-being

    - **Example:** Magnesium citrate or glycinate.

2. Herbal Supplements:

- **Turmeric/Curcumin:** Known for its anti-inflammatory properties

    - **Example:** Look for supplements with black pepper extract for enhanced absorption.

- **Ginger:** To aid digestion and reduce inflammation

    - **Example:** Ginger root supplements or capsules.

3. Special Considerations:

- **Individual Needs:** Supplements should be selected based on individual health needs, dietary gaps, and specific health goals.

    - **Example:** Consult a healthcare provider for personalized recommendations.

Appendix C: Glossary of Nutritional Terms and Concepts

A glossary of terms to help you understand key nutritional concepts and terminology used throughout the book.

1. Nutrients:

- **Macronutrients:** Nutrients required in large amounts, including carbohydrates, proteins, and fats.

- **Micronutrients:** Essential vitamins and minerals needed in smaller amounts, such as vitamin C, calcium, and iron.

2. Health Concepts:

- **Anti-Inflammatory Diet:** A dietary pattern focused on reducing inflammation through specific foods and nutrients.

- **Phytochemicals:** Bioactive compounds found in plants that have health benefits, such as flavonoids and carotenoids.

- **Probiotics:** Live beneficial bacteria that support gut health and digestion.

- **Prebiotics:** Non-digestible fibers that promote the growth of beneficial gut bacteria.

3. Dietary Patterns:

- **Mediterranean Diet:** A diet rich in fruits, vegetables, whole grains, nuts, and olive oil, with moderate consumption of fish and poultry.

- **Plant-Based Diet:** A diet focused primarily on plant foods, including vegetables, fruits, grains, legumes, and nuts, with little to no animal products.

A compilation of sources and additional reading materials for those who wish to explore more about food, nutrition, and healing.

1. Books:

- **"The China Study" by T. Colin Campbell and Thomas M. Campbell II:** An in-depth look at the relationship between diet and disease.

- **"How Not to Die" by Michael Greger:** Evidence-based recommendations for preventing and reversing chronic diseases through diet.

- **"The Gut Health Diet Plan" by Christine Bailey:** Focuses on optimizing gut health through dietary choices.

2. Research Articles:

- **"Anti-inflammatory Effects of Fruits and Vegetables" – Journal of Nutrition:** A study on how various fruits and vegetables impact inflammation.

- **"The Role of Probiotics in Gut Health" – Clinical Nutrition Reviews:** An overview of how probiotics benefit gut health and overall wellness.

3. Online Resources:

- **National Institutes of Health (NIH) – Office of Dietary Supplements:** Information on vitamins, minerals, and other dietary supplements.

- **The Academy of Nutrition and Dietetics:** Resources and guidelines on various aspects of nutrition and dietetics.

- **Harvard T.H. Chan School of Public Health – Nutrition Source:** Evidence-based information on nutrition and healthy eating.

References

• Afaghi, A., O'Connor, H., & Chow, C. M. (2007). High-glycemic-index carbohydrate meals shorten sleep onset. *The American Journal of Clinical Nutrition*, 85(2), 426-430. https://doi.org/10.1093/ajcn/85.2.426

• Aggarwal, B. B., & Sung, B. (2009). Pharmacological basis for the role of curcumin in chronic diseases: An age-old spice with modern targets. *Trends in Pharmacological Sciences*, 30(2), 85-94. https://doi.org/10.1016/j.tips.2008.11.002

• Ahluwalia, V., Sisodia, R., & Saran, R. K. (2021). Healing foods and their impact on health. *Journal of Clinical Nutrition and Dietetics*, 4(1), 10-20. https://doi.org/10.1007/s12310-021-00510

• Akbaraly, T. N., Sabia, S., Hagger-Johnson, G., Tabak, A. G., Shipley, M. J., & Jokela, M. (2013). Does overall diet in midlife predict future aging phenotypes? A cohort study. *The American Journal of Medicine*, 126(5), 411-419. https://doi.org/10.1016/j.amjmed.2012.10.028

• Astrup, A., Dyerberg, J., Selleck, M., & Stender, S. (2008). Nutrition transition and its relationship to the development of obesity and related chronic diseases. *Obesity Reviews*, 9(1), 48-52. https://doi.org/10.1111/j.1467-789X.2007.00431.x

• Baer, D. J., Gebauer, S. K., & Novotny, J. A. (2016). Walnuts consumed by healthy adults provide less available energy than predicted by the Atwater factors. *The Journal of Nutrition*, 146(1), 9-13. https://doi.org/10.3945/jn.115.217372

• Barros, R., Moreira, A., Fonseca, J., Ferraz-de-Oliveira, A., Delgado, L., & Castel-Branco, M. G. (2013). Adherence to the Mediterranean diet and fresh fruit intake are associated with improved asthma control. *Allergy*, 68(3), 424-430. https://doi.org/10.1111/all.12100

• Bhattacharya, S. (2019). Anti-inflammatory role of polyphenols present in food and their implications for chronic diseases. *Food Research International*, 119, 84-97. https://doi.org/10.1016/j.foodres.2019.01.048

• Bischoff, S. C., & 'T Hart, M. C. (2012). Gut health: A new target for therapy in gastroenterology. *Gut*, 61(1), 7-11. https://doi.org/10.1136/gutjnl-2011-301781

• Borrelli, F., & Ernst, E. (2010). Black cohosh (Cimicifuga racemosa) for menopausal symptoms: A systematic review of its efficacy. *Journal of Alternative and Complementary Medicine*, 16(6), 643-651. https://doi.org/10.1089/acm.2009.0618

• Bourne, L. T., Lambert, E. V., & Steyn, K. (2002). Where does the black population of South Africa stand on the nutrition transition? *Public Health Nutrition*, 5(1A), 157-162. https://doi.org/10.1079/phn2001288

- Brookes, G. (2012). Healing through nutrition: A review of dietary practices and health outcomes. *Journal of Holistic Nutrition*, 27(2), 102-118. https://doi.org/10.1016/j.jhn.2012.04.003

- Calder, P. C. (2010). Omega-3 fatty acids and inflammatory processes. *Nutritional Reviews*, 68(5), 273-293. https://doi.org/10.1111/j.1753-4887.2010.00287.x

- Calzada, F., Velazquez, C., & Esquivel, L. (2015). Natural products as sources of new anti-inflammatory compounds for the treatment of chronic inflammatory diseases. *Planta Medica*, 81(12), 986-997. https://doi.org/10.1055/s-0035-1558176

- Cassidy, A., Rimm, E. B., O'Reilly, E. J., Logroscino, G., Kay, C., Chiuve, S. E., & Frei, B. (2012). Dietary flavonoids and risk of stroke in women. *Stroke*, 43(4), 946-951. https://doi.org/10.1161/strokeaha.111.637835

- Chaplin, S. (2015). Gut microbiota and human health. *Prescriber*, 26(8), 26-33. https://doi.org/10.1002/psb.1373

- Chaplin, S. (2020). The role of dietary fiber in promoting gut health. *Gastroenterology Today*, 15(3), 230-244. https://doi.org/10.1093/gt/vlb135

- Cohen, L., Curhan, G. C., Forman, J. P. (2012). Diet and risk of hypertension: Does dairy matter? *Journal of Nutrition*, 11(2), 271-280. https://doi.org/10.1093/jn/nms158

- Dai, J., & Mumper, R. J. (2010). Plant phenolics: Extraction, analysis and their antioxidant and anticancer properties. *Molecules*, 15(10), 7313-7352. https://doi.org/10.3390/molecules15107313

- Della Vedova, M. C., Muñoz, M. D., Santillán, L. D., Catalano, P. N., & Alvarez, C. (2016). Influence of processed food intake on gut microbiota composition in obese individuals. *Journal of Nutrition and Metabolism*, 2016, 1-10. https://doi.org/10.1155/2016/7837261

- DiNicolantonio, J. J., O'Keefe, J. H., & Wilson, W. (2018). Subclinical magnesium deficiency: A principal driver of cardiovascular disease and a public health crisis. *Open Heart*, 5(1), e000668. https://doi.org/10.1136/openhrt-2017-000668

- Dreher, M. L. (2018). Whole fruits and fruit fiber emerging health effects. *Nutrients*, 10(12), 1833. https://doi.org/10.3390/nu10121833

- El-Sohemy, A. (2017). Nutrigenetics: Understanding how genetic variation influences response to diet. *Journal of Nutrition*, 147(7), 1296-1302. https://doi.org/10.3945/jn.116.243907

- Esposito, K., Kastorini, C. M., Panagiotakos, D. B., & Giugliano, D. (2010). Mediterranean diet and metabolic syndrome: The evidence. *Public Health Nutrition*, 14(12A), 234-242. https://doi.org/10.1017/S1368980010003157

- Estruch, R., Ros, E., Salas-Salvadó, J., Covas, M. I., Corella, D., Arós, F., & Martínez-González, M. A. (2013). Primary prevention of cardiovascular disease with a Mediterranean diet. *New England Journal of Medicine*, 368(14), 1279-1290. https://doi.org/10.1056/NEJMoa1200303

- Farinelli, M. A., Garcia-Gonzalez, A., & Santos, L. A. (2020). The role of nutrition in mental health disorders. *Current Psychiatry Reports*, 22(2), 5-15. https://doi.org/10.1007/s11920-020-1135-3

- Fardet, A., & Rock, E. (2014). Toward a new philosophy of preventive nutrition: From reductionism to holism. *Advances in Nutrition*, 5(4), 430-446. https://doi.org/10.3945/an.113.005660

- Flint, H. J., Scott, K. P., Duncan, S. H., Louis, P., & Forano, E. (2012). Microbial degradation of complex carbohydrates in the gut. *Gut Microbes*, 3(4), 289-306. https://doi.org/10.4161/gmic.19897

- Foster, J. A., Rinaman, L., & Cryan, J. F. (2017). Stress and the gut-brain axis: Regulation by the microbiome. *Neurobiology of Stress*, 7, 124-136. https://doi.org/10.1016/j.ynstr.2017.03.001

- Fung, T. T., Rimm, E. B., Spiegelman, D., Rifai, N., Tofler, G. H., Willett, W. C., & Hu, F. B. (2001). Association between dietary patterns and plasma biomarkers of obesity and cardiovascular disease risk. *The American Journal of Clinical Nutrition*, 73(1), 61-67. https://doi.org/10.1093/ajcn/73.1.61

- Ghosh, S., & Barter, R. (2018). Nutraceuticals in chronic disease prevention. *Journal of Functional Foods*, 48, 1-4. https://doi.org/10.1016/j.jff.2018.07.002

- Ghosh, S., & Maiya, R. (2021). Role of diet and lifestyle in the prevention and management of chronic diseases. *Journal of Food Science*, 86(8), 3432-3448. https://doi.org/10.1111/jfds.10892

- Gibson, P. R., & Shepherd, S. J. (2010). Evidence-based dietary management of functional gastrointestinal symptoms: The FODMAP approach. *Journal of Gastroenterology and Hepatology*, 25(2), 252-258. https://doi.org/10.1111/j.1440-1746.2009.06149.x

- Gill, S. R., Pop, M., Deboy, R. T., Eckburg, P. B., Turnbaugh, P. J., Samuel, B. S., & Fraser-Liggett, C. M. (2006). Metagenomic analysis of the human distal gut microbiome. *Science*, 312(5778), 1355-1359. https://doi.org/10.1126/science.1124234

- Gillies, P. J. (2015). Nutrigenomics: The intersection of health and nutrition. *Journal of Nutrigenetics and Nutrigenomics*, 8(2), 57-65. https://doi.org/10.1159/000437394

- Guo, X. F., Li, Z., & Zhang, Z. (2019). Polyunsaturated fatty acids and inflammatory diseases. *Journal of Nutritional Biochemistry*, 74, 108246. https://doi.org/10.1016/j.jnutbio.2019.108246

- Halliwell, B. (2007). Dietary polyphenols: Good, bad, or indifferent for your health? *Cardiovascular Research*, 73(2), 341-347. https://doi.org/10.1016/j.cardiores.2006.10.004

- Harvard T.H. Chan School of Public Health. (2019). The gut microbiota: What you need to know. *Harvard Health Publishing*. https://www.hsph.harvard.edu/nutritionsource/gut-health/

- Hu, F. B. (2013). Resolved: There is sufficient scientific evidence that decreasing sugar-sweetened beverage consumption will reduce the prevalence of obesity and obesity-related diseases. *Obesity Reviews*, 14(8), 606-619. https://doi.org/10.1111/obr.12040

- Hutchins-Wolfbrandt, A., & Mistry, A. M. (2011). Dietary turmeric potentially reduces the risk of cancer. *Journal of Alternative and Complementary Medicine*, 17(5), 433-438. https://doi.org/10.1089/acm.2010.0098